BARIATRIC FITNESS

For Your New Life

A Post-Surgery Program of Mental Coaching,
Strength Training, Stretching Routines
and Fat-Burning Cardio

Julia Karlstad *M.Ed., CSCS, SFN-ISSA*

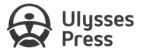

Published in the United States by:
Ulysses Press
P.O. Box 3440
Berkeley, CA 94703
www.ulyssespress.com

ISBN13: 978-1-61243-794-1
Library of Congress Control Number 2018930785

Printed in the United States by Kingery Printing
10 9 8 7 6 5 4 3 2 1

Acquisitions editor: Casie Vogel
Managing editor: Claire Chun
Editor: Lauren Harrison
Proofreader: Renee Rutledge
Indexer: Sayre Van Young
Front cover design: Justin Shirley
Photographs: © Bryan Nguyen
Interior design and layout: what!design @ whatweb.com
Production: Claire Sielaff
Models: Natalie Nelson, Matthew Martinez, Julia Karlstad
Contributing writer to Chapter 1: Laurel Dierking

Distributed by Publishers Group West

CONTENTS

INTRODUCTION

Fitness or exercise may seem like a simple component in the treatment phase of obesity, and thus it is often underemphasized and overgeneralized. You've probably heard your doctor say that you need to exercise more; maybe they've even told you to start walking, or suggested that you do some water aerobics or join a gym. And herein lies part of the problem: Where do you start? What exactly should you do? How long should you exercise? How many sets and reps do you do? The list goes on.

Although I applaud the physicians that encourage their patients to be physically active, exercise can be overwhelming for someone who is 50, 100, 200, or even 300 to 400 pounds overweight. And your doctor may not be the only one badgering you to exercise. Are your friends, family, and coworkers pushing you as well? You may have the best intentions to get moving, but you're unclear about what to do and have added this outside pressure from others. Maybe you've tried to exercise in the past, but every time you do you've experienced some of this: everything hurts, breathlessness, you feel weak, you injure yourself, you're not seeing results, you get bored, or simply give up. If you're already exercising, you might be at a point of frustration because you're not seeing progress with your weight loss. All of this may be weighing you down even more than your excess weight.

I've been working with the bariatric population for over a decade and what I've described here is a reality for many. *Bariatrics* is a medical term that deals with the causes, prevention, and treatment of obesity. This includes both medical and surgical weight loss patients! This book, *Bariatric Fitness for Your New Life*, will specifically address the exercise component of obesity. Most health care providers will acknowledge the fact that exercise is an important component for improved health and decreased body fat, but few take the time or simply don't have the knowledge base to provide a detailed program that will work for someone who is overweight to obese or has undergone bariatric surgery. Additionally, many of the mainstream fitness books, gyms, and programs are geared toward the moderately fit person with few to no medical conditions.

Bariatric Fitness for Your New Life is all about exercise for long-term sustainable weight loss. If you've had bariatric surgery, this book is for you. Even if you've never had the surgery (but maybe have contemplated it), and desperately want to lose weight and—more importantly—keep it off, this book is sure to guide you down a path of exercise and long-term weight loss success.

There is a science behind exercise for weight loss. I've spent most my health and fitness career helping overweight to obese people get fit and lose weight. Many of my clients have had bariatric weight-loss surgery, and through my education and experience, I have found the formula for long-term weight loss success, revealed in this book. It will inform, educate, and outline functional systematic exercise programs for those looking to lose the weight once and for all.

Designed to be a self-help tool, you can jump from chapter to chapter in this book in order to gain valuable information to help you with your weight-loss goals. However, I highly encourage you to read the first two chapters before skipping around. The first chapter, Get Your Mind Right, is incredibly powerful because if you're not in the right place mentally, you will struggle in your weight-loss journey. Chapter Two gives a detailed summary of how exercise will ensure that you keep the weight off. Once you've absorbed this knowledge, you'll be ready to dive into the workouts for weight loss: mobility work, cardiovascular training, strength training, and balance training. You'll also learn about bariatric nutrition and fueling for weight loss. Finally, any program is only as good as you are at following it, so methods for keeping yourself accountable will also be addressed.

Before you begin any exercise program, you should consult your physician as well as identify your restrictions and what type of movements you must avoid as pertains to your limitations and current health condition. If one of the exercises fosters a movement that could hinder or further injure your condition, be sure to avoid these exercises (i.e., if you have osteoarthritis in your knees, do not do lunges or high-impact activities such as running). Generally speaking, avoid or modify an exercise if you feel pain in a particular joint. Joint pain is not healthy pain. If the discomfort is in the muscle due to the activity itself, you are generally safe to continue (unless you have injured the muscle itself).

Chapter 1

GET YOUR MIND RIGHT WITH POSITIVE THINKING

The mind is one of the most powerful and influential components of the human body, and it plays a crucial role in weight loss. In fact, the average person has between 50,000 and 70,000 thoughts per day, or about 35 to 48 thoughts per minute (Davis, B., 2013). These thoughts and how you react to them can greatly impact your actions—or inactions— when it comes to successful weight loss. The constant chatter in your brain can prevent you from being present and self-aware, reduce mental clarity, alter your listening skills, and cause you to feel depleted and overwhelmed. Oftentimes we need to pause and think for a moment during stressful moments or when we are triggered by something. This "stop and think" practice allows you to be more mindfully aware of your thoughts, the emotions that arise from the situation, and, most importantly, decide how you will react. In other words, the best strategy for successful weight loss is to acknowledge what is happening, allow yourself to feel some discomfort, take some deep breathes, then respond to stress in a healthy manner, rather than going into default or autopilot mode, which may result in unhealthy patterns and consequently cause weight gain.

I often tell my clients, "If your mind isn't right, you will struggle with the weight-loss journey." So first and foremost, get your mind right! Doing so involves changing how you process thoughts and emotions throughout the day. You know what I'm talking about: that little voice that continually chatters, judges, and critiques the decision-making process. Sometimes it fills you up with positivity, and other times it fills your mind with negative and destructive messages. If you constantly look at life as a glass half full or are pessimistic about every situation, then you'll experience negativity in life! You are what you think. So it is critical to get your mind on a positive track. Do not get discouraged when you have setbacks because this is real life—there will be letdowns (a job change, loss of a loved one, an unexpected injury, getting sick, a bad day, and the list goes on). What's important is to understand that life events will happen, and it's *how* you choose to react to these events that matters.

EVALUATE AND REFLECT

All of this sounds great right, but it may be easier said than done—especially if you've had a history of failure with exercise and weight loss. I mean, it's not like this is your first rodeo. In fact, you're probably pretty darn good at losing weight; it's the keeping it off that may have been the challenge.

This time, I need you to spend a little time evaluating and reflecting on the past. Note your successful moments along with the not-so-positive ones. Jot down some things that may have either helped or hindered your success below:

What contributed to your weight-loss success?

What hindered your weight-loss success?

What contributed to your exercise success?

What hindered your exercise success?

....

....

....

Don't get stuck in the negative, but do spend a few moments evaluating what you could have done differently to be more successful in the negative moments. Similarly, hold onto what pushed you forward and allowed you to be successful with both your weight-loss and exercise initiatives. You may want to highlight those successful thoughts above.

This exercise will help you recognize the positive factors and potential roadblocks going forward. Understand, however, that you must let go of the negative and allow yourself to move forward and fill your mind with positive self-talk. In other words, be mindful; have a conscious awareness of your thoughts, feelings, and physical sensations in the present moment. This time you're committed to making this exercise and weight management thing a lifestyle change once and for all.

BE PRESENT AND MINDFUL

Be present in the moment, the now—be mindful! The better we master the art of being present and connecting with the here and now, the better we recognize our span of control and be at peace with knowing we need not worry about the past or the future. Eckart Tolle said it best in his book *The Power of Now: A Guide to Spiritual Enlightenment*:

> "*Give attention to the present; give attention to your behavior, to your reactions, moods, thoughts, emotions, fears, and desires as they occur in the present. There's the past in you. If you can be present enough to watch all those things, not critically or analytically but nonjudgmentally, then you are dealing with the past and dissolving it through the power of your presence.*"

The present moment is where your actions matter and this is the place you make change. This is where you can get your mind right and focus on positive thoughts. We can become aware of and practice gratitude, compassion, and self-acceptance in the present moment. This acceptance is an important catalyst in your weight-loss journey. It will help to focus your attention on what your strengths and goals are moving forward, rather than dwelling on shame or regret about what you feel you lack. But how do you get there? How do you practice gratitude for a situation that you are not happy or satisfied with? How do you accept yourself when you are ashamed or disappointed with your physical body? This mental and emotional dilemma can be the most challenging barrier to overcome, but it is not impossible. A paradigm shift in thinking will serve you well in changing the habit of negative self-talk into positive affirmation of yourself.

MEDITATION

Mindfulness and meditation are often mistakenly thought of as one in the same. They are, however, two separate practices. Meditation is an inward practice of reflection and contemplation that is restful and calming to the mind. Tigunait (2014) suggests that meditation is a practice, first and foremost. Specifically, it is the practice of becoming aware of our thoughts rather than turning them off. When we meditate and become aware of our thoughts, we can recognize our thought patterns, behaviors, beliefs, and positive or negative self-talk patterns, and determine if these habits are beneficial or not. We then can make a conscious effort to choose to no longer believe harmful thoughts or act on impulsive decisions and behaviors for the sake of repeating a habit.

Meditation can be done seated, lying down, walking, in silence, or even aloud with words or song. Meditation, like exercise, is a tool in your toolbox that not only helps you be more resilient on your weight-loss journey, but also offers the foundation for becoming more consistently present. The awareness cultivated during meditation is the foundation of mindfulness.

Recent research on the benefits of meditation show that individuals who meditate for as little as 10 minutes a day reduced their blood pressure, lowered perceived levels of stress, improved memory and cognitive function, and, arguably most importantly, reduced anxiety and improved overall perceived happiness (Horowitz 2010). Ultimately, meditation is a technique that can guide you into what this chapter is all about: getting your mind right. This is crucial for the success of your journey not only in reaching your weight-loss goals, but encouraging a mindset that is sustainable for you to be able to live a more fulfilling life.

MEDITATION PRACTICE

This visual meditation teaches the mind to become an objective observer of our thoughts and feelings, rather than letting those thoughts and feelings carry us off and enabling them to take over our mind. A river represents the mind, and we are an observer of the river sitting on its edge.

Find a quiet space where you will be uninterrupted for a period of time. I suggest starting with a realistic time goal of three to five minutes. Set a calm alarm to softly ring when your time is up, which will help you to not worry about time as you practice.

Sit comfortably on a chair, a cushion, or the floor; you can also choose to lie down, but do not fall asleep. Close your eyes. Direct your attention to your natural breathing pattern, just observing. Focus your attention on your breath and allow your mind to settle and relax. Work to deliberately focus on the present moment.

As you sit and breathe, picture yourself sitting on a river bank. Allow your mind to create the external environment and visualize the river in front of you. As is the premise of meditation, become a witness to your thoughts, feelings, and sensations that arise. The river you see is a visual representation of your thoughts. Simply sit back and watch the river flow by. Like the river, your mind will flow, bringing in thoughts, ideas, reminders, and stories. The idea is to watch them come and go. Focus on watching the river with a fixed gaze in your mind as you continue to breathe steadily.

If at any point you notice that your mind has wandered off, take notice that your mind has wandered. Express gratitude (rather than frustration) to yourself for realizing the distraction, and gently shift your attention back to the flowing river and your breath. Bring yourself out of the river and back onto the river bank, watching and observing, without attaching to a thought (e.g., jumping into the river).

Practice this for three to five minutes every day. As you become comfortable with meditating, gradually increase the meditation's duration to 20 minutes or more.

MINDFULNESS PRACTICE

Mindfulness supports a neutral, nonjudgmental witnessing of experience (Segal, Williams, and Teasdale 2002). This neutral witnessing includes an awareness of all of one's experiences, including thoughts, feelings, and body sensations. When you become mindful of your experience in the moment, you understand your response to sensations such as hunger, desire, or resistance to an activity (like exercise). This state of being mindfully present allows you to have control of what you do with the thought. You can act on your desire for the sweet treat and have it, or you can choose to not indulge in the desire that was merely triggered by a thought. Mindfulness gives you an opportunity to practice willpower and self-discipline in an objective way that is compassionate and empowering. Mindful practices can include:

1) Learning to become more aware of your posture throughout the day.

2) Practicing gratitude and appreciation for where you are on your journey, even if it is not where you *want* to be.

3) Recognizing and understanding stress, including the thoughts, emotions, sensations, and behavioral urges that build from an event (i.e., stressor) and may result in undesired behaviors.

4) Giving *one* task your full, undivided, and uninterrupted attention (e.g., washing the dishes, driving, or writing).

BREATH PRACTICE

The foundation of both mindfulness and meditation is one's breathing. The breath is the most underutilized tool that we already possess. Breathing is an autonomic body function like your heart beat or blinking; you do not have to consciously make an effort to do any of these. However, focusing on your breathing is the most direct way to quickly deactivate the chronic stress response within the body and activate the "rest and digest" state of the parasympathetic nervous system (PNS). This simple practice can lower heart rate and blood pressure, and slow down or even stop the production of cortisol, all of which have a major impact on weight loss and maintenance. Chronic stress plays a frighteningly large role in the health status of our population, and research shows this to be worsening. The good news is that breath is a tool that can be used to immediately counteract the dangerous effects of stress on our physical bodies.

Choose two consistent times during your day to stop, sit comfortably upright, and become aware of your breathing for one to two minutes. Find a quiet place without distractions. Commit every day for at least two weeks to taking just a couple of minutes to become aware of a few details of your breath. In doing so, you are practicing mindfulness while taking a short time out to develop healthier breathing habits. Begin by noticing a few details of the breath, including:

1) The length of your inhales and exhales. Are the inhales longer than the exhales, or vice versa?

2) The depth of your breath. Where do you feel that your breath stops in your body?

3) The location of your breath. Where do you feel the breath in the body and what body parts move when you breathe?

4) The quality of the in and out breaths. Are your breaths shallow, labored, forceful…or deep, effortless, smooth, etc.?

5) Are you breathing through your nose or your mouth?

6) Does anything tighten up on your body when you breathe?

As you practice and begin to recognize your own breathing habits, try and correct your breathing by:

1) Breathing in and out through the nostrils.

2) Making the exhales longer than the inhales.

3) Breathing deep into the belly, without lifting or straining the upper chest, shoulders, and/or neck muscles.

4) Relaxing completely on each exhale.

5) Increasing the volume of air you breathe in (bring more breath in with each inhale).

GOAL SETTING AND PERSONAL COMMITMENTS

Since you've made the decision to lose weight or even to have weight-loss surgery, it's imperative to set goals and personal commitments. Goals take some time to accomplish, while personal commitments are day-to-day or weekly accomplishments. Your goals will keep you focused on what you want to achieve in the long run, whereas your personal commitments or specific measurable action items will help you achieve and sustain those goals long-term. For example, maybe your goals are to lose 100 pounds and drop six pant sizes. Your personal commitments may look something like this: 1) eat a healthy breakfast every day; 2) limit sugar intake to no more than 25 grams per day; and 3) exercise four times per week. Notice that both the goals and personal commitments in this example are measurable so you can look back each week and check off your success with either a yes/no or how much. Jot down your goals and personal commitments below.

Goals:

....

....

....

....

....

Personal commitments (measurable action items that will help you achieve your goals):

....

....

....

....

....

....

Awesome! You've taken a big step toward improved health and fitness, and have set the foundation for your weight-loss success. Look back each week and check in with yourself to see how you're doing with your goals and commitments. This will help keep you on track. You've set a plan of what you want to achieve and how you're going to achieve it. If you stay disciplined and focused on the long-term goals and daily/weekly to-do items, you're giving yourself the tools to guarantee success.

ACCOUNTABILITY

Any plan or program is only as good as you're going to follow it; setting up accountability systems will be paramount to ensure you stick to your plan.

ASSESSMENTS

One of the first steps of an accountability system is to assess where you're at today. Do these self-assessments to gather good data about your health and fitness starting point.

Initial Assessment date:_____

ASSESSMENT	RESULT	REASSESSMENT RESULT
Weight (pounds)		
Waist Measurement (inches) *above the belly button*		
Hips (inches) *widest area of hips with feet together*		
Chest (inches) *across the nipple line; arms relaxed*		
Arms (inches) *mid-arm; between elbow and shoulder*	Right: Left:	Right: Left:
Legs (inches) *mid-leg; between hip bone and knee cap*	Right: Left:	Right: Left:
Blood Pressure		
Resting Heart Rate (bpm)		
1-minute sit-up, knee tap, or bench sit-up modification (total completed)		
1- minute full or modified push-ups (total completed)		
Wall squat or modified wall squat for time (seconds) *5 minutes maximum*		

You will need a scale, a tape measure, and a blood pressure cuff. If possible, find a friend or family member to help you perform all girth measurements. Record your result on the chart above. I encourage you to reassess every four to six weeks.

WEIGHT

Stand on a scale and record your weight in pounds.

NOTE: Be sure to always weigh yourself at the same time of the day, with no shoes and in similar clothing or no clothing at all. I also encourage you to weigh just once per week. It can be easy to get obsessed with the scale and we all fluctuate in weight throughout the day.

WAIST

Stand tall with feet hip-width apart. Find the belly button and place the end of the measuring tape to the side of the body while simultaneously bringing the measuring tape right above the belly button. Continue to extend and wrap the measuring tape evenly (parallel to the floor) around the entire body until the tape comes in contact with the starting point. Record measurement.

NOTE: Depending on your size, your belly button may be lower than your hips. If this is the case, pick a landmark (e.g., a mole or scar) on the mid-belly and measure the circumference as outlined above from that point. Make a note of the landmark as you'll use this point to reassess the waist circumference.

HIPS
Stand tall with feet together. Place the end of the measuring tape on the left hip. Extend and wrap the measuring tape evenly (parallel to the floor) around the entire body at the widest area of the hips until the tape comes in contact with the starting point. Record measurement.

CHEST
Stand tall with feet hip-width apart. Place the end of the measuring tape just to the right of the right nipple. Extend and wrap the measuring tape evenly (parallel to the floor) around the entire body until the tape comes in contact with the starting point. Record measurement.

NOTE: Depending on your size and age, your nipples may fall well into your mid-belly region. In this is case, measure the widest area of your chest. Make a note and use this point to reassess the chest circumference.

ARMS
Stand tall with feet shoulder width apart. Find the top of the shoulder and elbow to visualize and pinpoint the mid-arm. Place the end of the measuring tape at mid-arm. Extend and wrap the measuring tape evenly (parallel to the floor) around the entire arm (make sure your arm is relaxed, not flexed) until the tape comes in contact with the starting point. Record measurement. Repeat on the opposite arm and record measurement.

LEGS
Stand with a staggered stance and place all of your weight on the back leg. Find your hip bone and knee cap on the front leg to visualize and pinpoint the mid-thigh. Place the end of the measuring tape at mid-thigh. Extend and wrap the measuring tape evenly (parallel to the floor) around the entire thigh (make sure the leg is relaxed, not flexed) until the tape comes in contact with the starting point. Record measurement. Switch stance and repeat on the opposite leg.

BLOOD PRESSURE

Sit in a chair with your back resting against the back of the chair and feet shoulder width apart and in contact with the floor. Rest your hands in your lap. Wrap the blood pressure cuff around your upper left arm so that the hose of the cuff is in line with the inside of your elbow joint (the antecubital space). Take a few deep breathes, relax, breathe normally, and start blood pressure analysis. Take and record measurement.

RESTING HEART RATE (BEATS PER MINUTE)

This measurement is generally recorded with the blood pressure analysis. Record measurement.

1-MINUTE SIT-UP

The 1-minute sit-up targets abdominal muscular strength. This is a timed assessment. Start the timer as soon as you start your first sit-up. Count and perform as many sit-ups as you can in 1 full minute. Once the minute elapses, the assessment is complete. Record the number of sit-ups performed.

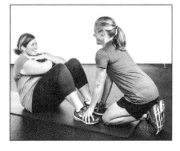

Sit-Up: Lie flat on the floor with knees bent at 90 degrees and feet flat on the floor. Have someone hold your feet or place your toes under a secure object (e.g., a couch). Cross your arms over your chest and keep them in contact with your chest throughout the exercise. Sit up until your elbows touch your thighs. Release back down to the floor until your shoulder blades touch the floor and then sit back up until the elbows touch the thighs again. Your head and shoulders do not need to come in contact with the floor each time, only your shoulder blades (i.e., upper back).

Knee Tap Modification: Instead of crossing your arms over your chest, extend your arms so that the palms of your hands are in contact with your thighs. Lift up until your fingertips touch the tops of your knees. Release back down until your shoulder blades touch the floor, and then lift back up until the fingertips touch the knees again. Your head and shoulders do not need to come in contact with the floor each time, only your shoulder blades.

Bench Sit-Up Modification: If you are unable to perform a full sit-up or knee tap, or you are unable to get down on the floor, perform a bench sit-up. Position the bench at an incline (the greater the incline the easier the sit-up). Lie down on the bench with your arms crossed over your chest and keep them in contact with your chest throughout the exercise. Sit up until your elbows touch your thighs. Curl the spine and release back down to the bench until your shoulder blades touch the bench. Immediately sit back up until your elbows touch your thighs again. Your head and shoulders do not need to come in contact with the floor each time, only your shoulder blades.

FULL PUSH-UP

The full push-up targets upper-body strength. This is a timed assessment. Start the timer as soon as you lower down for the first full push-up. Count and perform as many push-ups as you can in 1 full minute; record your score.

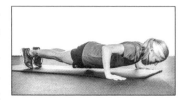

Push-Up: Get into a full plank position with your hands a little farther than shoulder-width apart and in line with the shoulders. Keep your back straight, core muscles tight, and lower your body down by bending the elbows. Lower until the elbows are bent at 90-degree angles and then push back up into your starting full plank position.

Knee Push-Up Modification: If you are unable to perform a full push-up, do a modified push-up from your knees. Get into a modified plank position with your hands a little farther than shoulder-width apart and in line with the shoulders. Your knees will be down and in contact with the floor. Follow the instructions for a full push-up.

WALL SQUAT

The wall squat targets your lower-body strength. Record the length of time you can hold the position with good form, no longer than 5 minutes.

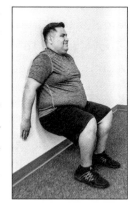

Stand with your feet shoulder width apart against a secure wall. With your heels positioned about 1½ feet away from the wall, slowly slide down the wall until your knees are bent at 90 degrees and your thighs are parallel to the ground. Your feet should be stacked under your knees. Press your back into the wall, engage your core, and hold that position as if you're sitting in a chair without the chair.

Wall Squat Modification: Perform a wall squat as indicated above, but only bend the knees to 120 degrees.

ACCOUNTABILITY SYSTEMS

The next step in setting yourself up for success is to build your accountability network. Create systems that will help keep you on track and focused on your goals and personal commitments. There are numerous professionals that can contribute to your success. Not sure where to start or whether or not to seek professional help? Ask yourself these questions:

1) What date did you have your weight-loss surgery? If it was less than six months ago, you should be having monthly follow-up visits with your weight-loss surgeon and his or her team of health care providers. You'll still see your weight-loss surgeon after six months, just less frequently.

2) Are you struggling with your nutrition? Eating too little, eating too much, not eating the right foods, not sure of what foods to be eating? Seek out a registered dietitian or nutritionist. They can help set up a dietary accountability system.

3) Are you exercising? Not sure if your exercise program is complementing your goals? Have you struggled in being consistent with your exercise? Personal trainers can be great motivators and accountability coaches. They'll set up a game plan to ensure your workout regimen complements your health and weight-loss goals.

4) Do you have a physical injury or health complication? Maybe a physical therapist (PT) is the best place to start with your exercise program and then you can transition to a personal trainer. The PT can aid in the recovery of your injury or health condition, and then you'll need to make sure and follow through with the exercises they give you.

5) Do you find yourself struggling with your mind? Are you stuck in your unhealthy habits and can't seem to stop gravitating toward them? Don't hesitate to seek out a mental health professional if this is something you still struggle with.

Your friends and family can also be excellent support systems and accountability tools. Surround yourself with positive people and tell them what you're doing. Then they can help check in with you to see how it's going. Share your goals and personal commitments with your family. Since your immediate family will be participating in your journey by sharing meals with you, maybe going to doctors' appointments with you, and even exercising with you, it will be very important to let them know what exactly you want to accomplish. Get a friend or coworker to start exercising with you. Another healthy tactic might be having a coworker share healthy lunches with you. Make sure they understand what a healthy meal looks like for you, as it might be very different from what they are eating and that's OK—especially if you've had weight loss surgery and they haven't. Educate them about the surgery so that they know what you're going through.

Digital devices, apps, and tech gadgets can be wonderful tools for exercise and weight-loss success. Two free apps that I frequently recommend to my clients are MyFitnessPal and LoseIt, which will assist in tracking your daily nutrition and activity. Similarly, there are numerous fitness tech gadgets that can boost your workout accountability. I'm a big fan of the Polar heart rate monitor as well as Fitbits, and, depending on the model, they can track daily activity, calories burned, intensity, distance traveled, sleep, and more.

Your accountability system may look something like the Accountability Wheel below:

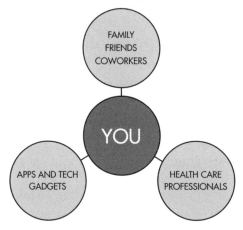

Remember that you are the center of your accountability wheel—you're in the driver's seat and you have control over your destiny. You don't have to have all the other spokes attached to your wheel, or maybe you have additional accountability spokes not covered. The key is to have accountability systems (i.e., spokes) in place because the more spokes you have, the stronger the wheel, the greater the momentum, and the better chance you'll have for success. Your program is only as good as you're going to follow it, and most of us need accountability systems in place to keep us focused on the desired outcome.

Chapter 2

GET YOUR BODY RIGHT PHYSICALLY AND NUTRITIONALLY

Believe it or not, exercise is not the most important factor in losing weight, although it is critical for long-term weight-loss success and weight management (i.e., keeping the weight off). So, I want you to start thinking of exercise as insurance for not only your health, but also your weight loss efforts. The more you invest (i.e., exercise) the stronger and more reliable the insurance.

Let's break this down a bit further. Losing weight is not an easy task, and keeping it off can be an even bigger challenge. Exercise absolutely plays a part in helping you lose weight, so start now or continue if you're already working out. Just understand that your nutrition combined with weight-loss surgery will initially have a greater impact on your weight loss. If you haven't had weight-loss surgery and are only changing your exercise habits without changing your diet, chances are that you will not lose as much weight as you'd like. The good news is that if you've adopted a sound exercise program into your life, keeping the weight off once you've lost it becomes a much smaller challenge. In fact, you're almost guaranteed to keep the weight off as long as you're balancing nutrition with consistent, regular exercise. And this is why exercise is critical, and thus your insurance, for long-term weight management.

ANATOMY AND METABOLISM

Maybe you have this idea that the weight-loss surgery is going to be your golden ticket for weight loss. I mean, that's why you had it, right? To ensure this weight comes off once and for all?

As you know or may have experienced first-hand by now, weight loss surgery changes the anatomy of your gastrointestinal system. Bariatric surgery, such as the gastric sleeve, gastric bypass, and laparoscopic adjustable gastric banding, changes the stomach and digestive system, which in turn causes the body to change how it processes both macro and micronutrients or all food, including vitamins and minerals. Your weight-loss surgery team will teach you how to eat according to these anatomical changes. Remember that regardless of which bariatric surgery procedure you have, the surgery itself is a tool! In other words, you must allow this tool to work; you can't just expect magic to happen. A hammer doesn't work unless you have a nail and someone to use the hammer to pound the nail in. Similarly, your long-term weight loss success will depend on many factors such as nutrition, exercise, behavioral changes, and more. If you put in the work of exercising, making healthy dietary choices, and keeping your mind right, your weight loss surgery will be that golden ticket to success.

Metabolism slows with age and it also slows with weight loss—we all battle this natural physiology. Maybe you're thinking, "My metabolism is already slower than molasses, and now you're telling me it's going to be even slower?" Yes, and that's why you must exercise to help speed up your metabolism to reverse this trend. Your metabolism slows down anywhere from 2 to 10 percent per decade depending on your age and your activity level. The biggest reason for the decline is not just that you're aging, but that people tend to be less active as they age, have more fat mass than when they were younger, and subsequently have less lean muscle mass. This should help motivate you to latch onto this exercise thing once and for all! It truly is your only saving grace to all the other things that slow down your metabolism. The bottom line is, the fitter you are, the higher your metabolism. That's why fit people tend to be leaner; they are much better fat burners, even when they're sleeping.

Now it's time for you to be a better fat burner, and to ease the struggle of keeping the weight off and be able to enjoy a few of life's simple pleasures without the guilt. Ultimately, I'd like to you to get to the point where you can enjoy that burger, glass of wine, or dessert and feel like you're living rather than cheating. Stop correlating your food with your integrity. That's defeating and self-sabotaging and can derail your healthy mind. We do need to reward ourselves at times—maybe once a week or a couple of times a month. It will also be important to find several non-food items to reward yourself with, but occasionally it's okay to have the not-so-healthy food or drink. Just be mindfully aware of what you're doing, never binge, and understand that this is in part why you exercise. It's okay to have these things here and there. We all do it. The key is moderation, and only if it's coupled with regular exercise can you avoid the weight gain associated with the treats.

EXERCISE AS INSURANCE

The reason I say that exercise is insurance is because if you do the work, you'll be investing in your health and weight-loss goals. In order to have security in your insurance, you must invest! With exercise, the premiums aren't dollar amounts; rather they are paid with each workout. And the more workouts, the better the insurance. You see, exercise is the magic pill for improved health and long-term weight loss. It has been confirmed that exercise will do the following:

- decrease anxiety and depression
- decrease mortality
- improve cholesterol
- improve flexibility and balance
- improve immune system
- improve self-confidence and your social life
- improve sleep
- improve vascular circulation
- increase cardiovascular health
- increase energy, allowing you to enjoy activities with friends and family
- increase lean muscle mass
- increase strength
- lower blood pressure
- lower blood sugar and triglycerides
- prevent osteoporosis
- relieve stress

Truly amazing—and this list isn't even complete. There's not a single medication on the market that can give you that many benefits in one fell swoop with no negative side effects. The key to reaping the benefits though is that you consistently do the work. Once again, we're talking about lifestyle change. This isn't something you'll only invest in for a short period. Because despite all the healthy benefits of exercise, once you stop exercising, the negative impact happens quite quickly. And before you know it, all the investment effort you put in through blood, sweat, and tears will be quickly lost.

So in short, exercise must be an ongoing thing in your life. In other words, you can't stop exercising. And if you haven't started, start today! Just like you wouldn't let your insurance lapse, you can't let your exercise lapse.

NUTRITION

As you tackle the exercise component of your healthy lifestyle, always be vigilantly in tune with your nutrition. Nutrition will always be the most important component of weight loss, and your nutritional needs will change depending on where you are in your weight-loss journey, especially for weight-loss surgery patients. Here's a snapshot of what your nutrition is going to look like the first year pre- and post-weight-loss surgery.

1 to 2 week pre-op diet: This diet will vary depending on your surgeon, but many programs will put you on a high-protein liquid diet pre-operatively. Sugars, caffeine, and carbonated beverages will also be eliminated. This plan is designed to decrease the amount of fat around key organs such as your liver and spleen, making it easier to navigate the anatomy during surgery. It also facilitates weight loss and starts your healthy dietary habits. Daily caloric intake will vary depending on your size.

1 to 2 weeks post-op diet: The first week post-op will be all liquid, and then you'll graduate into pureed foods, along with liquids and protein drinks. Sugars, caffeine, and carbonated drinks are off-limits. Daily caloric intake will range between 400 and 800 calories depending on your size.

3 to 6 weeks post-op diet: This period is about protein shakes and soft foods, and will incorporate a reintroduction of soft high-protein foods such as egg whites, soft cheeses, yogurt, cooked or pureed vegetables, avocados, and fish. Daily caloric intake will range between 400 and 800 calories depending on your size.

6-plus weeks post-op diet: Start to introduce solid foods back into your diet. You do not get to eat whatever you want, but you'll start to feel like you're eating more normally again. Your solid food diet should still be high-protein and consist of proteins, vegetables, some grains, and virtually no refined sugars. I suggest you introduce one new solid food at a time to give your body time to react and adjust to the new food. Daily caloric intake will continue to range between 400 and 800 calories for the first three months post-operatively. As you lose weight and get in better shape, your body may require more calories past the three-month mark. Talk to your bariatric doctor and/or dietitian or nutritionist for specific caloric and food type recommendations. Generally, 12 months post-op you'll be taking in 1,000 to 1,200 calories daily. This value can rise depending on your metabolism and overall activity level. Ultimately, I like to see patients get to a daily caloric intake of about 1,500 calories or more for weight maintenance. This is more than achievable through proper nutrition and regular exercise.

Supplements: Bariatric surgery dramatically decreases your body's ability to absorb nutrients, causing malabsorption and vitamin and nutrient deficiencies. As a result, weight-loss surgery patients will be required to take the following supplements as recommended by their doctor: multivitamin, iron, and calcium citrate (don't take iron and calcium at the same time of day, as they compete with each other's absorption).

Water: Get in at least 64 fluid ounces per day. Don't drink any liquids with meals (ideally no liquid 30 minutes before a meal and wait 60 minutes after a meal). Also, avoid drinking anything out of a straw (to avoid unwanted air in the stomach).

One potential side effect of bariatric surgery is dumping syndrome. This occurs when you eat too many sugary foods, refined carbohydrates, or high-fat foods. The stomach will not fully break the food down before dumping it into the intestines. This can cause cramping, nausea, sweating, increased heart rate, diarrhea, and vomiting—essentially, you're going to feel sick. Dumping syndrome can occur in gastric bypass, duodenal switch, and gastric sleeve patients, and doesn't occur with every patient, but you'll want to avoid it at all costs.

Now be prepared to struggle a bit in making these changes. You've spent a majority of your life creating and reinforcing unhealthy eating habits. Although you're changing your habits, some of those old habits are programmed into your brain, and it will take time to deprogram the bad and reprogram the good. This is why the mental component of this process is so important (refer to Chapter 1 for more insight on this topic).

EATING AND EXERCISE

Since weight loss is your main objective, it can be easy to fall into an "I'm not hungry" or "I shouldn't eat" thought process. The weight-loss surgery itself will cause you to be hungry far less often than you ever used to be; this is due to the anatomical change combined with the major dietary change. It's not a bad thing if your hunger cravings were a struggle before! However, this can cause problems in the long run if you don't pay attention, especially as it relates to your workouts.

Depending on the time of day you work out, it may not be necessary to eat prior to exercise. But it's very important to get something in your body within 45 minutes after you work out. This may seem strange or even counterproductive. You just burned a good number of calories, why would you want to consume those calories right after your workout? Well, because you need to train your body to be an efficient fuel burner and also ensure the body is tapping into the right calories at the right time. You have a 45-minute window to refuel after a workout and in turn reap the most benefit from the exercise and recover optimally. I'm not suggesting you eat a big meal, but after exercise, do get 100 to 300 calories that's approximately half protein and half carbohydrate. One of the main goals with post-op exercise is to maintain the lean muscle mass and target the fat mass. In other words, preserve your muscle and lose the fat.

The body predominately burns two fuel sources: fat or carbohydrates. Protein is not an efficient fuel source and the body will only tap into protein for fuel when it's in a state of starvation or there aren't sufficient calories available. So, with adequate caloric intake, specifically amino acids (which are the building blocks for protein), the body will use carbohydrates or fat for energy. This is ultimately the goal: to burn fat! And so taking in a higher-protein diet will be vital to force the body to tap into the fat cells and facilitate weight loss, especially during the first year after weight-loss surgery. Diet plays an important role in targeting the fat calories you want to burn to reach your goals and achieve long-term sustainable weight loss.

Carbohydrates are your body's preferred source of fuel because they are the most accessible and the easiest to break down. Carbohydrates are found as glucose in the blood stream and glycogen (stored glucose) in your muscles and liver. Whenever you first start exercising, no matter what form of exercise, you'll initially start to burn these carbs, adenosine triphosphate (ATP), to be exact, which is the simplest form of carbohydrate (remember the Krebs cycle from biology class?).

As you continue to exercise, you'll also tap into fat calories for fuel. You burn fat best at low to moderate intensities, and you'll burn the largest percentage of fat calories through cardiovascular exercise. But remember there is a science here: It takes longer to break down and metabolize fat, thus your best bet to burn more fat is to exercise at low to moderate intensities. Keep in mind that the body utilizes oxygen to burn fat and this is essentially why you'll burn more fat doing cardiovascular exercise—because you must have oxygen to burn fat. Since cardio or aerobic exercise essentially means "with oxygen," this form of exercise will require fat metabolization.

As you increase the intensity of your cardio, you'll start to tap into more and more carbs for fuel because you need more energy, and the body can get to the carb fuel more quickly. Intense exercise will ultimately force the body to tap into glycogen stores and eventually you'll reach a point where you'll be burning 100 percent carbohydrates. When you get to this level of intensity, you have now transferred over into the anaerobic system (i.e., without oxygen) and thus you are no longer burning fat. Now the more fit you are, the better you burn fat at higher intensities and for longer durations. This is why fit people tend to be leaner: They have trained their bodies to be better fat burners, while exercising and even when they are sleeping. This is also why sound nutrition and the timing of that nutrition will help maximize fat loss. Sounds like good motivation to get your body right through diet and exercise!

Chapter 3

MOBILITY WORK

Mobility as it relates to your body is the ability to move. And I would propose that everyone has a mobility goal to move freely, independently, and without restriction or pain for as long as possible as they age. One method for achieving mobility is to move or exercise, kind of like the saying that "in order to get energy you must burn energy." Movement is quite similar because if you want to increase movement, you must get moving. There are several specific exercise techniques or programs that can improve your mobility and, most importantly, reduce pain, speed recovery, and prevent injury. I refer to these programs and techniques as mobility work. This chapter outlines four different mobility programs, including easy-to-follow pictures and descriptions for each movement. Start incorporating some of these programs into your weekly routine and you'll immediately feel the benefits of doing mobility work.

NOTE: Many of these exercises can be performed from a seated position, so if your joints hurt when you stand or you get too fatigued to stand for long periods of time, feel free to do them from a seated position.

RANGE OF MOTION

Range of motion (ROM) is how far you can move a joint in different directions, and the goal is to be able to move each joint freely through its entire ROM. Performing these exercises daily or even a couple of times a day will help keep your joints functional and flexible.

Always warm up for at least 5 minutes before getting into your actual workout. The ROM routine below can act as a warm-up, and may be better than a traditional warm-up such as walking slowly or riding a stationary bike for 5 minutes because these exercises will prepare *all* of your joints for movement. Always keep breath work (see page 12) in mind while performing these exercises; the breath work will play a factor in your mental health and keep you focused and present in the exercise. Depending on what your fitness level is, this ROM routine may be your weekly workout for the first couple of weeks and/or can be used as a daily meditation/relaxation routine. If you're short on time, pick four or five of the exercises to perform versus the entire routine.

CAUTION: If you suffer from a neck condition (e.g., degenerative disc disease, stenosis, or fused or herniated discs in the cervical spine), some of these neck mobility exercises may be contraindicative for your neck. Check with your doctor before performing these movements.

Front to Back

Target: neck mobility ◉ This exercise may also be performed from a seated position.

1 Stand tall with your feet hip-width apart and your arms at your sides. Look straight ahead. Inhale and slowly bring your chin toward your chest until you feel a stretch at the base of your neck.

2 Exhale and slowly rotate your head up and back until you feel a stretch across your throat.

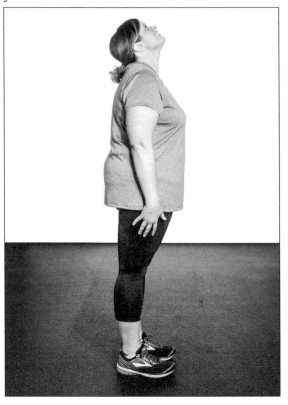

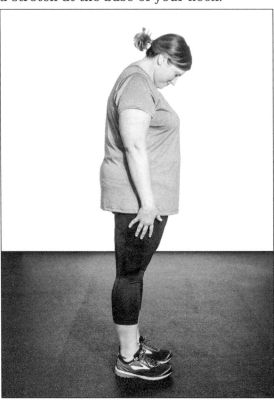

Continue for 10 repetitions.

Side to Side

Target: neck mobility ◎ This exercise may also be performed from a seated position.

1 Stand tall with your feet hip-width apart and your arms at your sides. Look straight ahead. Inhale and slowly bring your left ear toward your left shoulder until you feel a stretch across the right side of the neck.

2 Exhale and bring your right ear toward your right shoulder until you feel a stretch across the left side of your neck.

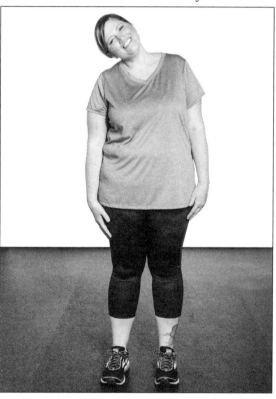

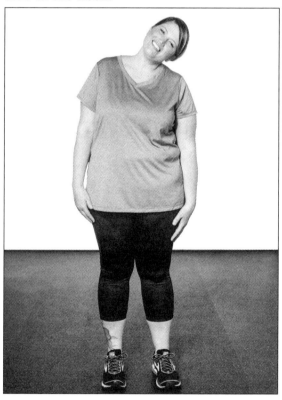

Continue for 10 total repetitions.

Wrist Circle

Target: wrist mobility ◎ This exercise may also be performed from a seated position.

1 Sit on a chair with your feet hip-width apart and your forearms outstretched and resting on your knees with your hands relaxed. Slowly rotate your wrists in one direction for 10 repetitions.

2 Switch directions for 10 more repetitions.

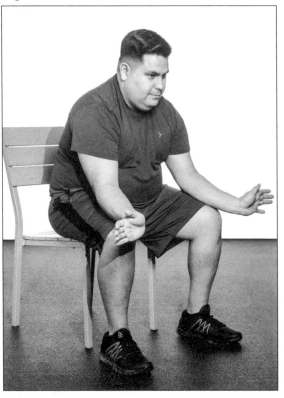

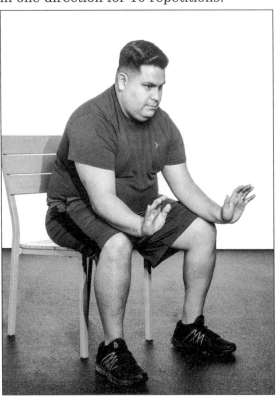

Dump the Sand

Target: shoulder mobility ◎ This exercise may also be performed from a seated position.

1 Stand tall with your feet hip-width apart and your arms stretched out to your sides with palms facing up. Exhale and slowly rotate your shoulders until your palms are facing down and back behind you. Think of dumping sand out of your hands.

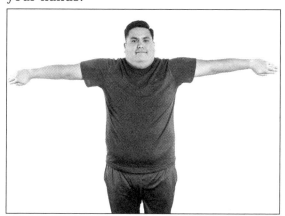

2 Inhale and slowly rotate your shoulders back around until your palms are facing up.

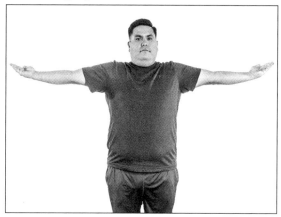

Continue for 10 repetitions.

Overhead Clap

Target: shoulder mobility ◉ This exercise may also be performed from a seated position.

1 Stand tall with your feet hip-width apart. Stretch your arms out to your sides parallel to the ground with your palms up.

2 Inhale and slowly bring your arms up and overhead until your palms touch or clap one another, or until you feel discomfort.

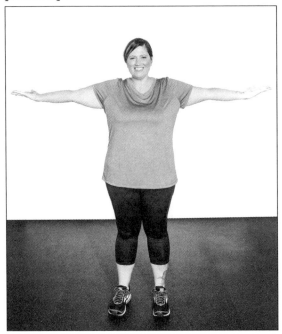

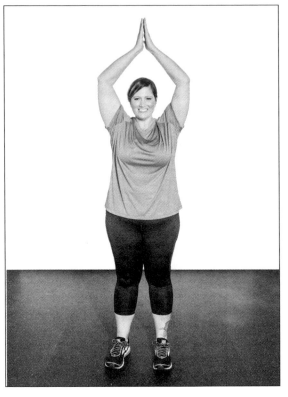

Exhale and return to the starting position.

Continue for 10 repetitions.

Trunk Rotation

Target: core mobility

1 Lie on your back on the floor with your knees bent at about 90 degrees, feet flat on the ground, and hands at your sides.

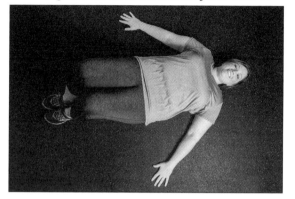

2–3 Keep both shoulders flat on the ground as you slowly rotate both knees over to your right side as far as your body will allow (ideally the leg closest to the floor will touch the floor). Your feet will rotate and come off the floor, but be sure to keep the legs bent and stacked on top of one another. Take a breath.

On your next inhale, bring your knees up back through the starting position and over to your left side. Take a breath.

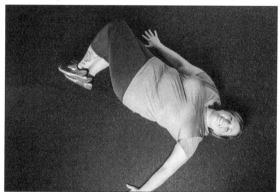

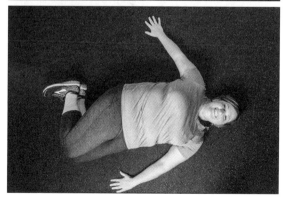

Continue for 10 total repetitions.

Hip Rotation

Target: hip mobility

1 Stand tall with your feet hip-width apart in a neutral position, and use a chair or wall if needed for balance. Inhale and slowly bring the left leg up so that the knee is at a 90-degree bend with the thigh parallel to the ground.

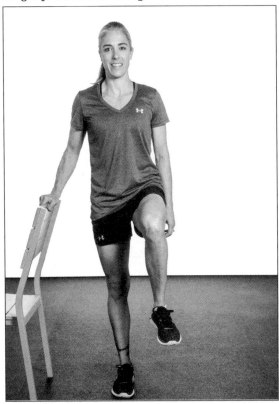

2 Rotate the leg out and away from the body in a circular motion.

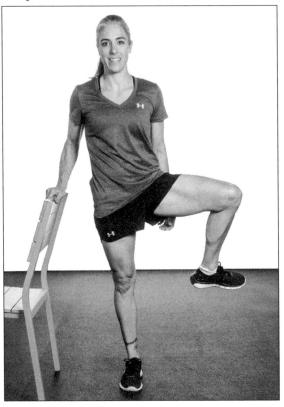

Exhale and bring the leg back down to its starting position.

Continue for 10 repetitions and then repeat on the right leg.

Leg Swing

Target: hip mobility

1 Stand tall with your feet hip-width apart in a neutral position, and use a chair or wall on your left side for balance during the exercise.

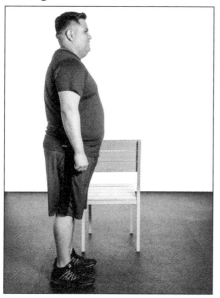

2–3 Slowly swing the right (outside) leg up and out in front of you while maintaining a slight bend in the knee of the leg you're moving. Keep a rhythmic inhale/exhale breathing pattern throughout the ROM.

Let the right leg fall and swing back behind your body.

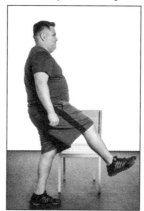 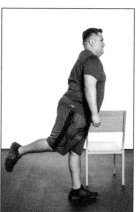

Continue for 10 repetitions and then turn around and repeat on the opposite leg.

Wide-Stance Side to Side Rock

Target: hip mobility

1 Stand tall with your feet wide apart, toes forward, and hands palms down and in contact with the upper part of your thighs.

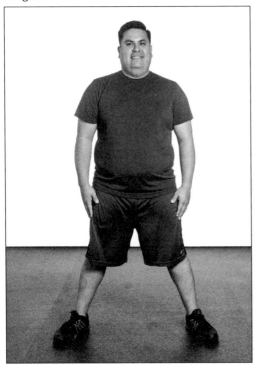

2 Inhale and slowly bend the right knee and lean to the right; allowing the hands to slide down toward your knees. Keep your back flat (do not round it) and sit back into the movement so that your right knee is bent about 30 degrees and the left leg is straight, with the knee fully extended.

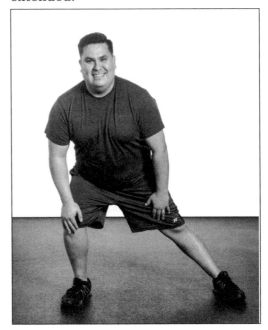

Exhale and slowly transition to the opposite side so that your left knee is bent about 30 degrees and the right leg is straight. Continue to maintain a flat back and keep both feet in contact with the ground.

Continue for 10 repetitions; back and forth is 1 repetition.

Leg Extension

Target: knee mobility

1 Sit tall in a chair with your back straight and in contact with the back of the chair; keep your knees bent with both feet flat on the floor.

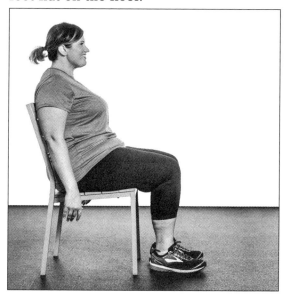

2 Inhale and slowly lift and extend the right leg to full extension.

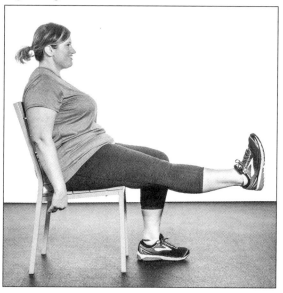

Exhale and bring the right leg back to its starting position.

Continue for 10 repetitions, and then repeat on the opposite leg.

Leg Curl

Target: knee mobility

1 Stand tall with your feet hip-width apart in a neutral position, and use a chair or wall if needed for balance.

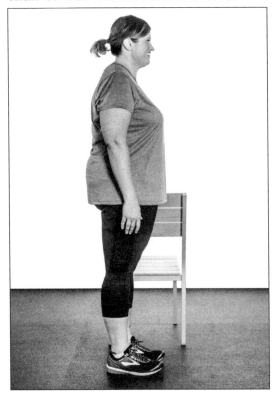

2 Inhale and slowly lift and curl the right leg back behind you so that the heel of your right foot is moving up away from the floor and directly behind you as far as you can bend it.

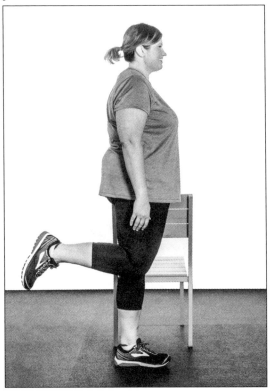

Exhale and bring the foot back to its starting position.

Continue for 10 repetitions, and then repeat on the opposite leg.

Ankle Circle

Target: ankle mobility

1 Sit tall on a mat or bench with your back straight and a yoga block propped under your left calf.

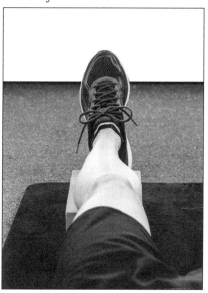

2 Slowly move your left foot in a clockwise circular motion: in (inversion), downward (plantar flexion), out (eversion), and up (dorsiflexion).

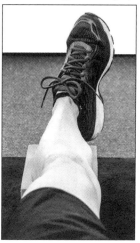
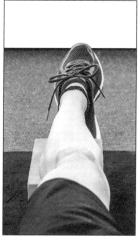

Continue for 10 repetitions, and then switch directions so that you are moving the ankle counter-clockwise; repeat on the opposite ankle in both directions.

Ankle Alphabet: This variation is similar to ankle circles, but instead of moving your foot in a circular motion, you'll simply spell or "draw" the alphabet with your toes. Start with A and end with Z before switching ankles.

STRETCHING

It is important to have good flexibility, or the ability to move your joints "pain free" in their intended range of motion. This is very similar to the Range of Motion program (page 29) as far as the definition is concerned, but the programming is different in that you'll be holding static (or stationary) positions versus moving the joint in a continual range of motion. Having good flexibility ultimately helps you move freely, prevents injury, and prevents muscle imbalances.

Before you stretch, it is best to warm up with 5 to 10 minutes of light activity. The ROM program in this book can serve as a warm-up, or you may want to walk slowly or do another form of a total-body cardiovascular movement at a low intensity.

While stretching, don't bounce; in other words, hold a static stretch of one position and breathe throughout your stretches. If you feel pain, back off; you'll want to feel a light pull, but don't stretch to the point of pain, which can result in something called a reverse reflex (causing the reverse effect of what you're trying to accomplish, when the muscles to tighten up rather than stretch out). Hold each stretch for a minimum of 10 seconds and a maximum of 90 seconds. Try to do this flexibility routine daily. If you're short on time, pick a handful of the exercises to perform versus the entire routine, and always stretch the muscles you worked out after your exercise routine.

It may help to purchase a stretching or yoga strap to aid in performing some of these stretches. If you don't have a strap you can always use a belt or a resistance band with a handle to assist as well.

CAUTION: If you suffer from a neck condition (e.g., degenerative disc disease, stenosis, fused or herniated discs in the cervical spine), some of these stretches may be contraindicative for your neck. Check with your doctor before performing these stretches.

Forward and Back

Target: neck ◉ This exercise may also be performed from a seated position.

1 Stand tall with your feet hip-width apart. Slowly bring your chin toward your chest while placing your hands on the back of your head to assist in the stretch. You'll feel a stretch at the base of your neck. Hold for 10 to 90 seconds.

2 Cup your hands over one another and bring your knuckles underneath and in contact with your chin and elbows down in front of your chest.

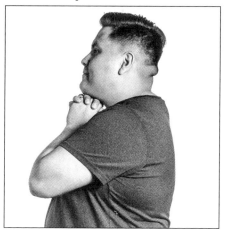

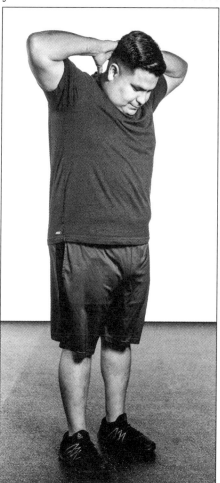

3 Slowly rotate your head up and back while keeping your hands directly under your chin and gently pushing up to assist in the stretch. You'll feel a stretch across your throat. Hold for 10 to 90 seconds.

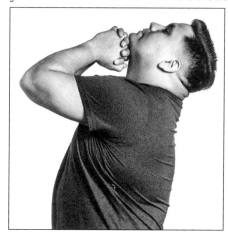

Side to Side with Bent Elbow

Target: neck ◉ This exercise may also be performed from a seated position.

1 Stand tall with your feet hip-width apart. Clasp your right wrist behind your back with your left hand, and pull your right arm so that the left elbow is sticking out to the left side of your body.

2 While holding the starting position, slowly rotate your left ear toward your left elbow until you feel a good stretch across the right side of your neck. Hold for 10 to 90 seconds.

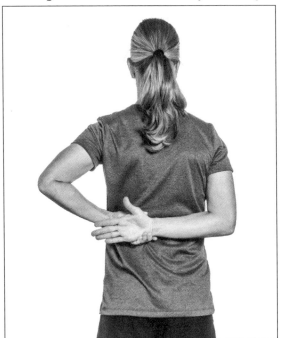

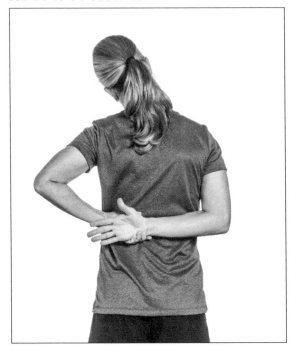

Repeat on the other side.

Forearms

Target: forearm ◎ This exercise may also be performed from a seated position.

1 Stand tall with feet hip-width apart. Extend your right arm out in front of you and place your left hand over top of your right hand; use your left hand to slowly pull your right-hand fingers down toward the floor and toward your chest until your wrist is bent approximately 90 degrees or more. Hold for 10 to 90 seconds.

2 Now bring your right fingers up toward the ceiling using your left arm to help pulling the fingers back toward your chest until your wrist is bent about 90 degrees. Hold for 10 to 90 seconds.

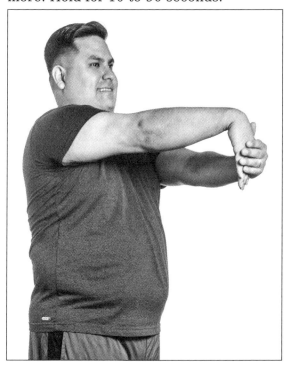

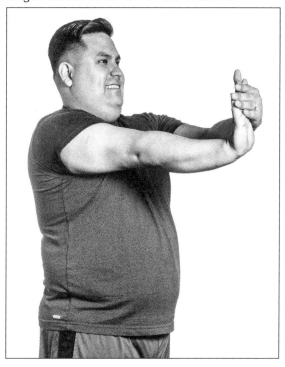

Repeat on other side.

Shoulder Rotation with Outstretched Arms

Target: shoulder

1 Stand tall with feet hip-width apart. Stretch your arms in front of you with your palms together.

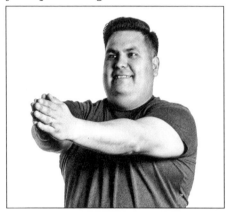

2 Find a soft object (e.g., a bed, end of a bench, or back of a couch) and place the back of your left hand on the object and then simultaneously begin to bend over at the waist.

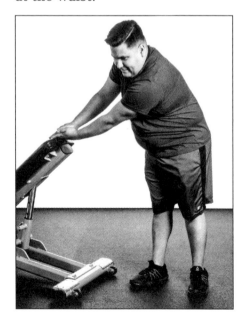

3 Now rotate down and away from the object you've placed your hands on (ideally past a 90-degree bend in your waist) until you feel a good stretch across the right shoulder. Hold for 10 to 90 seconds.

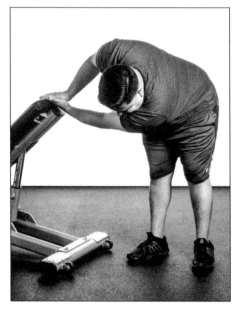

Repeat on other side.

Doorway Stretch

Target: chest and biceps

1 Find a doorway and place your palms on the doorframe anywhere below shoulder height.

2 Slowly walk forward through the doorway keeping your arms extended and in contact with the doorframe until you feel a good stretch across your chest and bicep muscles. Hold for 10 to 90 seconds.

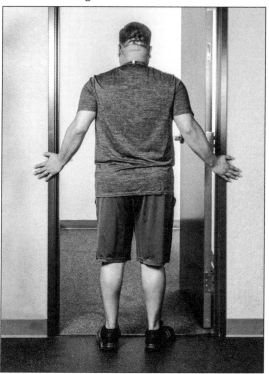

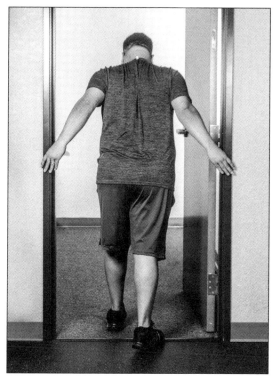

Triceps Wall Stretch

Target: triceps

1 Stand facing a wall with your right foot forward, about 6 inches from the wall, and left foot back. Bring the right elbow up and place the back of your arm (triceps) on the wall.

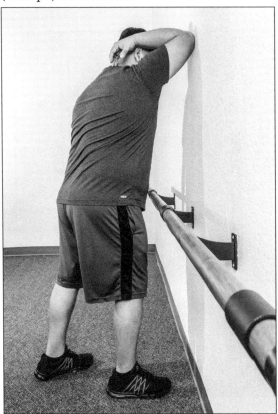

2 Slowly lean into the wall until you feel a good stretch on the back of your arm. Hold for 10 to 90 seconds.

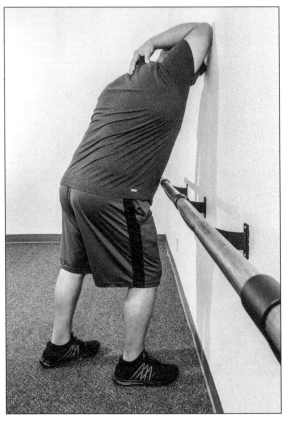

Repeat on the opposite side.

Upper Back Stretch

Target: upper back

1 Stand and grasp a secure object with both hands (preferably a rail or pole that is positioned anywhere between waist and shoulder height).

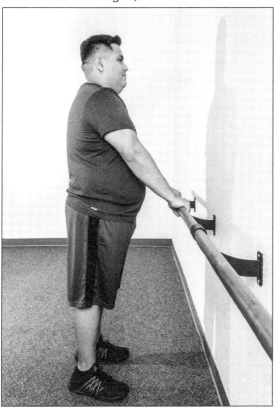

2 Step back and slowly bend forward at the waist; simultaneously let your head drop between your arms while maintaining a grip on the rail. Allow your shoulders to rotate forward and arch your upper back slightly until you feel a stretch across your upper back between the shoulder blades. Hold for 10 to 90 seconds.

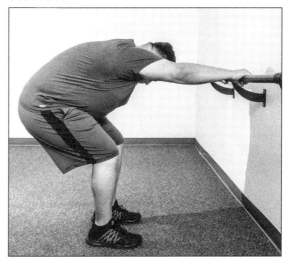

Low Back Stretch

Target: low back

1 Sit tall on the front half of the chair with feet flat on the floor and legs close together. Place your left hand on the outside of your right thigh and grasp the chair behind you with your right hand.

2 Slowly rotate to the right and place your right hand behind you while using your left hand to help push you into a rotation. As you rotate, look over your right shoulder and hold this position for 10 to 90 seconds.

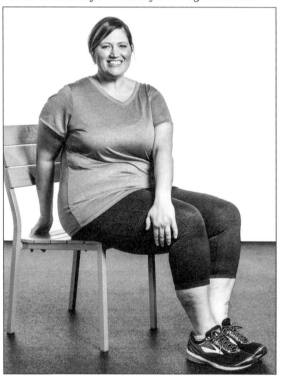

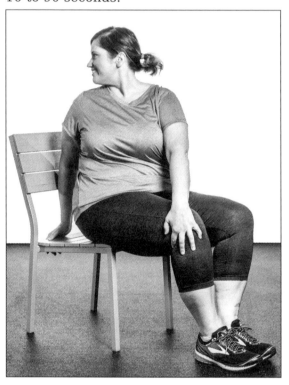

Repeat on the opposite side.

Hip Flexor Stretch

Target: hips

1 Stand tall in a wide split stance with your right foot in front of the left, toes facing forward, right knee slightly bent, and hips square to the front (use a secure object for balance if needed).

2 Slowly lean forward, bending your right knee and keeping your torso upright. Lean your upper body back slightly until you feel a stretch across the left hip flexor (upper thigh and across the front of your hip on the back leg). Hold for 10 to 90 seconds.

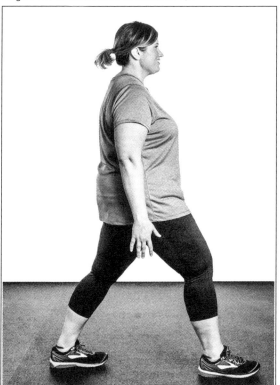

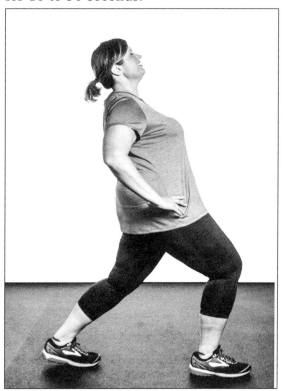

Repeat on the opposite side.

Piriformis Stretch

Target: hips

1 Sit tall on the front half of a chair with feet flat on the floor.

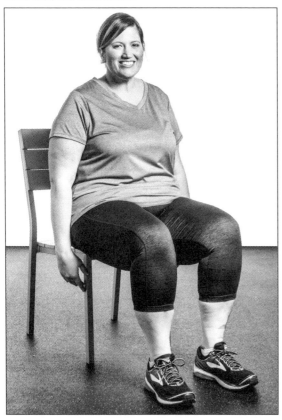

2 Place your right foot on your left knee. Leading with your chest, slowly lean forward and simultaneously press down on your right knee until you feel a stretch across the right outer hip. Hold for 10 to 90 seconds.

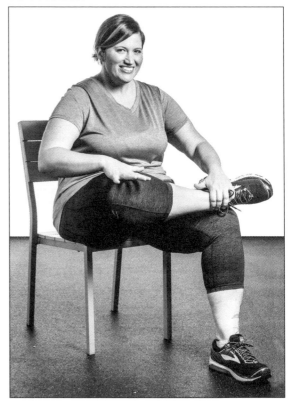

Repeat on the opposite side.

Quadriceps Stretch

Target: thighs (quadriceps)

1 Stand tall with your feet shoulder-width apart. You may want to stand next to a secure object for balance.

2 Slowly lift your right leg by bending your right knee, and grasp your right ankle with your right hand.

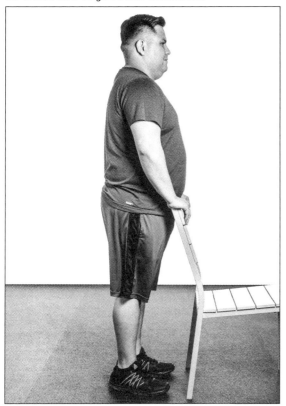

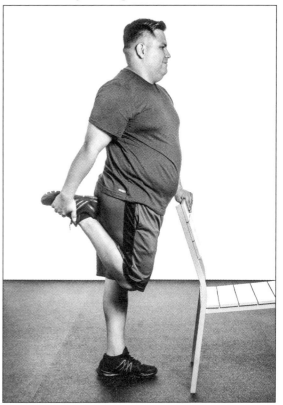

Slowly allow the knee to point toward the floor while the heel of your foot is positioned directly behind your butt. Stand tall until you feel this stretch across the top of your right thigh and hold for 10 to 90 seconds.

Repeat on the opposite side.

Modified Quadriceps Stretch

Target: thighs (quadriceps) ◉ If a chair is too high for your current flexibility, use a small stool or step to place your foot on instead of a chair.

1 Stand tall with your feet shoulder-width apart next to a stationary object and with a chair behind you. Place the right toe/top of your foot on the chair behind you while both hands grasp the secure object for balance.

2 Slowly push your hips forward while simultaneously leaning back slightly until you feel the stretch across the top of the right thigh. Hold for 10 to 90 seconds.

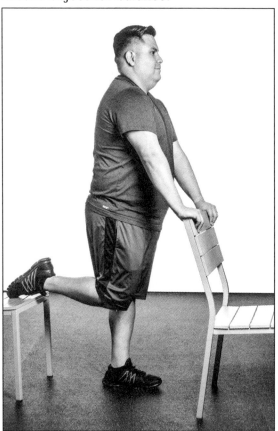

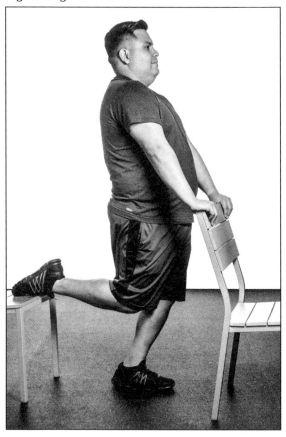

Repeat on the opposite side.

Seated Hamstring Stretch

Target: hamstrings

1 Sit on a bench, couch, or bed (firmer surfaces are better) with your right foot outstretched and your left foot flat on the ground.

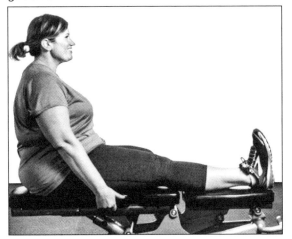

2 Square your shoulders up toward the foot of the outstretched leg and slowly lean forward; lead with your chest and keep your back relatively straight. Reach your hands toward the outstretched foot. Hold for 10 to 90 seconds.

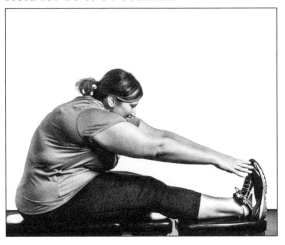

Repeat on the opposite side.

Adductor Stretch

Target: adductors

1 Stand next to a secure object with your feet wide and place your hands on a secure object.

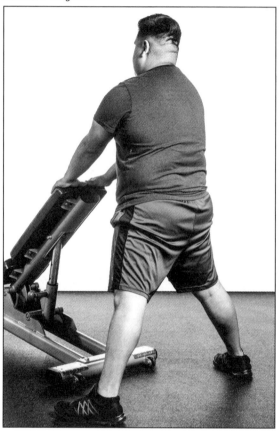

2 Slowly lean to your right by bending the right knee, pushing your hips back (i.e., leaning back into the stretch by pushing the right hip out and back), and keeping the left leg straight until you feel a stretch on the inside of your left leg (adductors). Hold for 10 to 90 seconds.

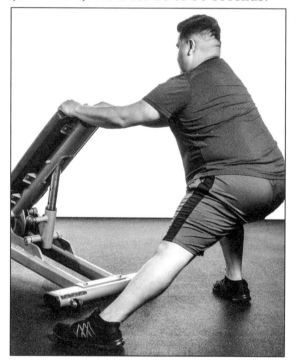

Repeat on the opposite side.

Abductor/IT Band Stretch

Target: abductors

1 Lie on the floor on your back (supine). Slowly bring your right leg straight up in the air while keeping the left leg flat on the floor.

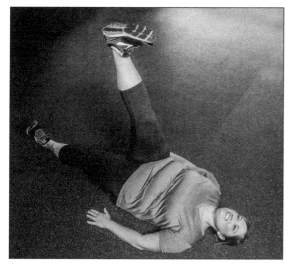

2 Slowly drop the right leg over and across your body while keeping both shoulders flat on the ground. Hold for 10 to 90 seconds.

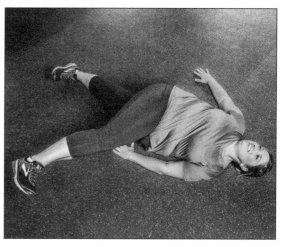

Repeat on the opposite side.

Glute Stretch

Target: glutes

1 Lie on the floor on your back (supine). Bring your right knee up toward your chest and outside of your rib cage.

2 Grasp your right knee with both hands and pull the knee down and toward the floor. Hold for 10 to 90 seconds.

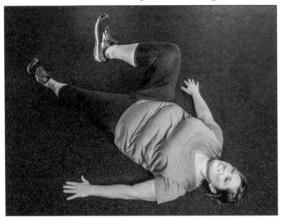

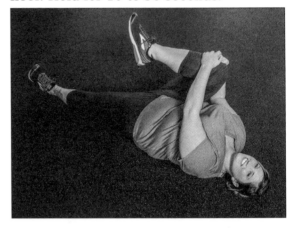

Repeat on the opposite side.

Anterior Tibialis/Shin Stretch

Target: anterior tibialis/shins

1 Sit tall in a chair with your right ankle on your left thigh. Grasp your right toes with your left hand.

2 Slowly pull the right foot back until you feel a stretch across the shin. Hold for 10 to 90 seconds.

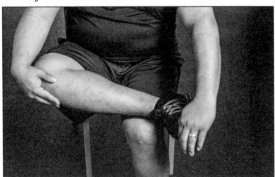

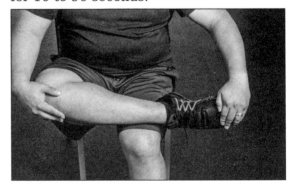

Repeat on the opposite side.

Gastrocnemius Stretch

Target: calves

1 Stand tall with feet shoulder-width apart facing to a wall, and place both palms on the wall at shoulder height.

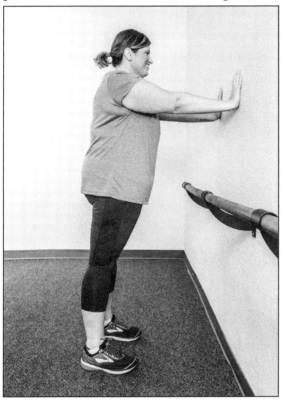

2 Bring your right foot back behind you so that the right leg is straight with the toes forward and your left foot is facing toward the wall with the left knee bent. Slowly lean forward into the wall until you feel the stretch on the back of the right calf; try to keep the right heel in contact with the floor. Hold for 10 to 90 seconds.

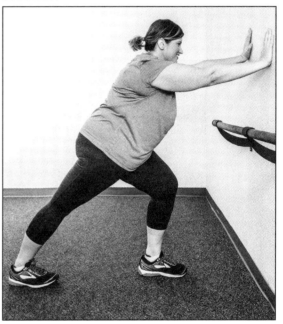

Repeat on the opposite side.

Soleus Stretch

Target: calves

1 Stand tall with feet shoulder-width apart facing a wall, and place both palms on the wall at shoulder height. Place your feet in a staggered stance with the right foot behind the left by about 3 inches.

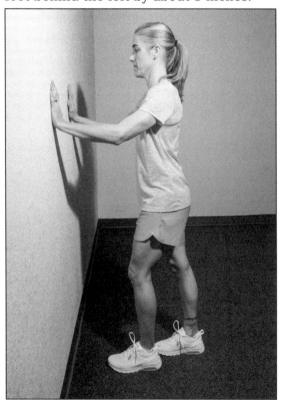

2 Slowly bend both knees while focusing on the right knee and leaning forward by placing your weight into your toes. You'll feel this stretch into the deep calf muscle (soleus) and all the way into your Achilles tendon (the very bottom portion of the back of your ankle) on the right foot. Hold for 10 to 90 seconds.

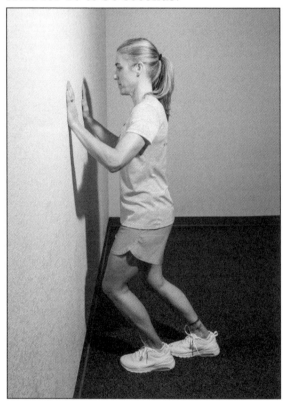

Repeat on the opposite side.

YOGA

Yoga is one of the best forms of exercise that not only incorporates range of motion and stretching, but also challenges your balance, facilitates strength, and helps center and clear your mind. It took me nearly 35 years before I started to do yoga on a regular basis, and wow was I missing out on the many benefits. If I had practiced yoga earlier in my life, I'm confident it would have prevented many of the sports-related injuries I have suffered over the years (ACL reconstruction, plantar fascia tear, numerous ankle sprains, ganglion cyst removal surgery, and arthritis, just to name a few). For now, however, yoga allows me to manage previous injuries, speed up the recovery of my workouts, decrease pain, and improve mobility. Yoga also gives me a tremendous amount of mental strength and wellness due to its emphasis on mind/body connection.

Don't wait for as long as I did to reap all the powerful benefits of yoga! Start today with this gentle beginner yoga program. Yoga is an excellent complement to any exercise routine. I suggest you start doing yoga once a week and then build up to two to three times a week, or practice it daily.

CAUTION: If you suffer from a neck or back condition (e.g., degenerative disc disease, stenosis, fused or herniated discs in the spine) some of these yoga poses may be contra-indicative for your spine. Check with your doctor before performing these yoga poses.

Mountain Pose/Tadasana

Target: posture awareness

1 Stand tall with your feet close together and your big toes touching. Find a neutral position with your body so that your chin is parallel to the ground, your shoulders are back and down, your chest is slightly out, and your arms are reaching toward the ground with the palms facing forward and fingers outstretched.

2 Gently inhale and draw your lower abdominal muscles in while filling your lungs with air.

3 Maintain the position and exhale. Repeat for 3 to 5 breaths.

NOTE: This is the starting point for most standing poses. It is a great resting/meditation pose and a great tool for posture awareness. With each breath imagine your rib cage expanding outward while your chest expands up. Focus on the posture and breath while maintaining this stable pose. To challenge yourself, try doing this pose with your eyes shut.

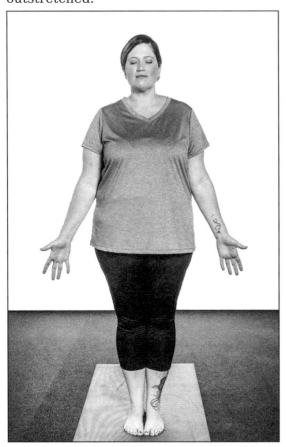

Standing Side Bend

Target: obliques

1 Begin in Mountain Pose (page 62) Slowly bring your arms up and overhead until they are outstretched with palms facing toward one another and touching.

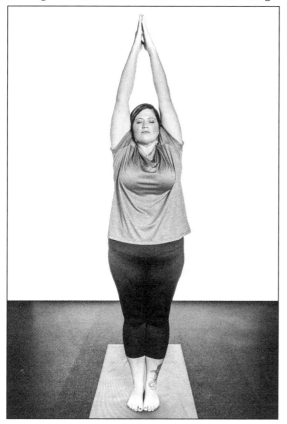

Inhale and try to keep the arms fully extended with your biceps close to your ears and reach your fingertips to the ceiling. Hold this position for 3 to 5 breaths, elongating your spine with each breath (imagine creating space between the vertebrae).

2 Inhale and slowly reach to the right with your arms still overhead and shift your hips to the left. You are creating a crescent moon with your body and will feel a stretch across the left side-body. Hold this side stretch for 3 to 5 breaths.

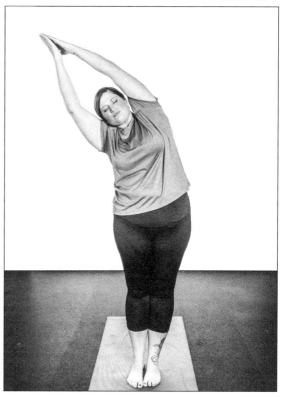

With the next inhale, slowly come back to center and slowly move the arms over and to the left. Shift the hips to the right until you create a stretch across the right side-body. Hold for 3 to 5 breaths.

Standing Forward Bend/Uttanasana

Target: low back/hamstrings

1 Begin in Mountain Pose (page 62). Exhale and slowly bend over at the hips (not the waist) while letting your arms extend down toward the floor.

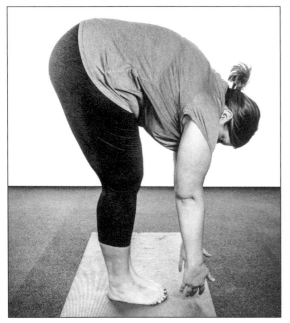

2 Cross your arms and simply let the head hang down between the arms. Hold for 3 or 4 breaths.

If your flexibility allows, extend the arms and bring your fingertips to the floor or allow the palms to rest on the floor. You can even wrap the hands behind the ankles and pull the forehead to the knees or shins for a deeper stretch. Hold for 3 to 4 breaths.

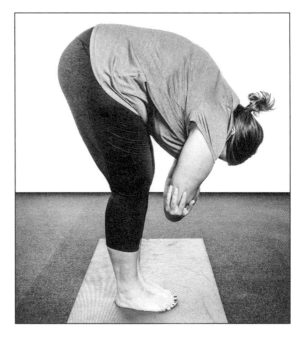

NOTE: With each inhalation in the pose, try to lift your sit bones toward the ceiling and lengthen the torso with each exhalation. Allow yourself to release a little more into the forward bend with each breath.

Chair Pose/Utkatasana

Target: legs/low back/core

1 Begin in Mountain Pose (page 62). Slowly reach your arms up and overhead with palms facing one another and shoulder-width apart.

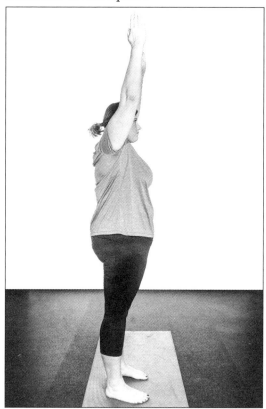

2 Inhale and slowly bend the knees and sit back and down so that the thighs are as close as parallel to the floor as possible, as though you are sitting in a chair. Your knees will come over your ankles some, but make sure you're not putting your weight into your knees. Instead, sit back into your heels, allowing your quadriceps, hamstrings and glutes to support you in this pose. Hold for 3 to 5 breaths.

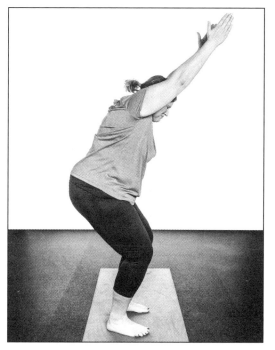

NOTE: Chair pose helps strengthen the feet, ankles, legs, shoulders, and back. It also stretches out the shoulders and chest and stimulates the diaphragm and internal organs.

Cat Cow/Marjaryasana Bitilasana

Target: back/spine mobility

1 Begin on your hands and knees with the back straight or in table-top position. Make sure your knees are stacked under your hips and your hands are directly under your shoulders, with the hands flat on the floor. Keep the head positioned so that you have a neutral spine (i.e., your head is straight out from your back, eyes looking down).

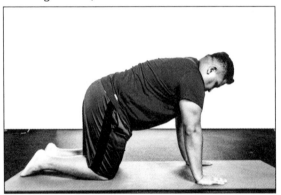

2-3 Slowly inhale and lift your sit bones and chest up toward the ceiling while your belly sinks toward the floor and the head lifts and looks straight forward (this is known as the cow pose).

Transition by exhaling and moving your spine so that the back lifts and rounds up toward the ceiling while your head drops down toward the floor (this is known as cat pose).

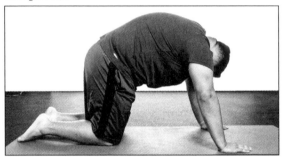

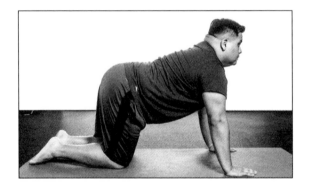

Repeat this movement for 5 repetitions so that you are always inhaling through the cow position and exhaling through the cat position.

NOTE: If you are unable to get down to the floor or cannot kneel, you can perform this exercise standing with the hands on a chair. Once you are in this modified table-top position, do the same exact movements as outlined above.

Bird Dog

Target: low back/core

1 Begin on your hands and knees with the back straight or in table-top position. Make sure your knees are stacked under your hips and your hands are directly under your shoulders, with the hands flat on the floor. Keep the head positioned so that you have a neutral spine (i.e., your head is straight out from your back, eyes looking down).

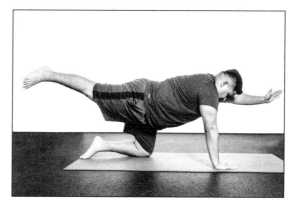

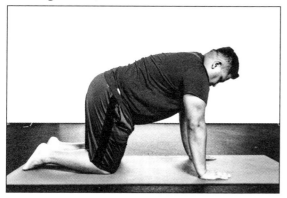

2 Inhale and slowly stretch your left arm out in front of you with the palm facing in; simultaneously lift the right leg up and stretch that leg so that both the left arm and right leg are parallel to the floor. Draw your belly button to your spine as you perform this motion and keep your back straight and squared up to the floor.

Exhale and return to starting position. Repeat on the opposite side.

Alternate side to side for 5 repetitions on each side while maintaining rhythmic breath work.

NOTE: If you are unable to get down to the floor or cannot kneel, you can perform this exercise standing with the hands on a chair. Once you are in this modified table-top position, do the same exact movements as outlined above.

Downward Dog/Adho Mukha Svanasana

Target: total-body stretch

1 Begin on your hands and knees with the back straight or in table-top position. Make sure your knees are stacked under your hips and your hands are directly under your shoulders, with the hands flat on the floor. Keep the head positioned so that you have a neutral spine (i.e., your head is straight out from your back, eyes looking down).

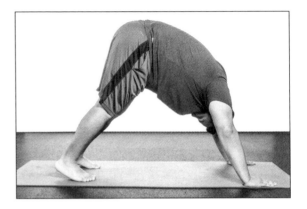

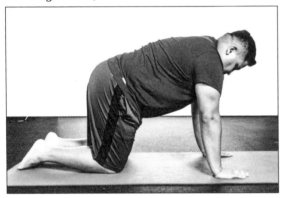

2 Begin to slowly lift the sit bones up toward the ceiling, bringing your knees off the floor and pushing against the mat through the palms of your hands. Allow your head to drop between the arms and push your chest toward your knees. You want to feel somewhat light in your hands and as if someone is taking your tailbone and pulling it by a string up toward the ceiling. Tighten your upper thighs and hold for 3 to 5 breaths.

NOTE: This recognizable yoga pose offers a total-body stretch. Initially, you might have to keep the knees bent and let the heels be lifted off the floor. You can even pedal the legs back and forth by bending the knee and pushing the heel down and then switching sides, but ultimately the goal is to push both heels into the mat and fully extend the legs. Also, you can perform this exercise standing with the hands placed on a sturdy chair. Once you are in this modified position, do the same exact movements as outlined above.

Upward Dog/Urdhva Mukha Svanasana

Target: core stretch

1 Begin by lying face down (prone) with the tops of your feet in contact with the floor. Place the palms of your hands on the floor so that the heels of your hands are in line with your rib cage.

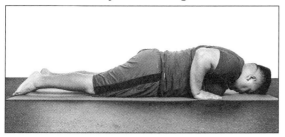

2 Inhale and slowly push your upper body up off the floor using your low back and upper body muscles. Do not allow your shoulders to creep up into your ears; this is a common mistake and will happen if you allow your weight to rest into your wrists.

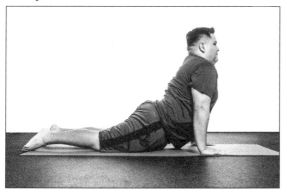

3 Tighten your thighs, and pull the abdominal muscles toward the back of your spine as you exhale; your feet may even lift off the floor a bit. Hold for 3 to 5 breathes.

NOTE: This is a powerful pose for the upper body and offers mobility and strengthening of the low back along with an incredible stretch of the abdominal muscles. If you feel like you don't have enough upper-body or low-back strength to get into this pose, it may be best to use a bolster, firm pillow, or a couple of yoga blocks to assist in achieving this position. Place your bolster so that the bottom of it is at your pelvis and the top is under your chest. Perform the exercise as outlined above. The bolster will offset the distance you're lifting your body weight, making it easier to get into the position.

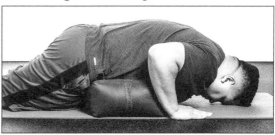

Child's Pose/Balasana

Target: low back and shoulders

1 Begin on your hands and knees, and move your arms out in front of your shoulders, palms down. Put your big toes together and keep the knees wide.

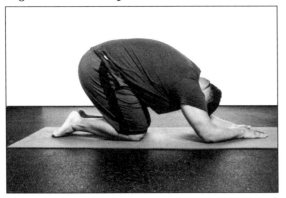

2 Exhale and slowly sit back into your heels. This is a resting position and can also be used anytime you feel you need a break during your yoga session or simply need a little more time before transitioning into the next pose.

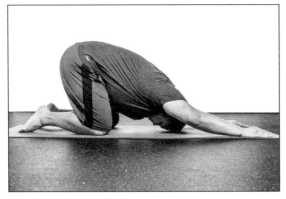

You can also bring the arms down along your side with the palms facing up and place the forehead into the ground.

NOTE: You may not be able to bend your knees or bring your shoulders all the way out overhead for a traditional child's pose. If so, simply place a bolster behind your legs, between the hamstrings and the back of your ankles, to decrease the range of motion in your shoulders and knees for this position. If you don't have a bolster, you can use a yoga mat or towel. All other positioning will remain the same.

Corpse Pose/Shavasana

Target: restoration, relaxation and breath work

The Position: Lie on your back (supine) with your arms at your sides with palms up and the legs positioned so the heels are as wide as the yoga mat. Let the feet fall open and feel your muscles relax with a sensation that you're melting down into the floor with each exhale.

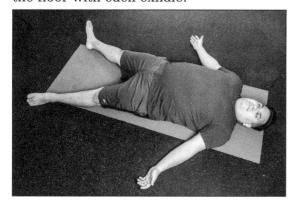

NOTE: This is a completely conscious pose with the goal of being fully awake yet completely relaxed. It is generally done at the end of a yoga routine and is one of deep restoration. It can also be an ideal pose in which to practice meditation. Despite how easy it may look, many people find it's much harder to master Shavasana than any of the rest. Shavasana is a practice of relaxing one body part at a time, slowly releasing the tension of each muscle and letting go of one thought at a time. Acknowledge your thoughts, but don't hang onto them; let them go and become fully alive and aware of your breath throughout this pose. Every single exhale should release a little more tension and bring you into a little deeper state of relaxation.

MYOFASCIAL WORK

Myofascial release (MFR) is an effective technique where you apply pressure on the connective tissue that covers the muscles (myofascial tissue). Fascia is found throughout the body, and "myo-" refers specifically to the muscle. The human body endures a tremendous amount of physical, mental, and emotional work every day. This repetition may cause stress, dehydration, injury, strain, or inflammation, which can ultimately cause pain through sensitivity and tightening of the myofascial tissue. The tightening of the tissue, if left untreated, may lead to more inflammation, increased muscle tightness, and/or decreased oxygen to that area.

Some of the main benefits of MFR include:

- Facilitating movement in your lymphatic system, which helps improve immune response

- Increased blood flow

- Keeping the muscles long and functional

- Reduced muscle soreness and faster recovery time

Pain usually originates in specific areas called "trigger points" or hot spots. However, just because you experience pain in a particular area doesn't mean that this is the region that needs to be treated. For example, pain around the knee, hips, or hamstrings could be a result of tight glutes or even back muscles. Thus, when you do MFR, work in broad areas. Additionally, don't spend more than 1 to 2 minutes per area; take enough time to perform 3 to 5 passes or rolls over the targeted area. In other words, don't roll one area for too long. Also, don't ever roll over a joint (e.g., if you're rolling out your thighs, don't roll over the knee). If you find a particular spot that is more painful or needs more work, hold the myofascial tool in that position for 45 to 60 seconds. This direct pressure will allow the muscles to relax a bit.

There are countless myofascial release tools that you can use to practice this therapy. This program uses two of the most popular tools: a foam roller and a myofascial release ball (trigger point ball). The foam roller is a long cylinder used to apply direct or indirect pressure to the muscles and relieve muscle tension. A trigger point ball offers similar benefits, but can create a deeper tissue release due to the smaller size and different positioning you can gain with the ball. As you practice these exercises, you'll feel tender/trigger points. Use a combined technique of holding and rolling over these areas. Choose an MFR tool that works for you and start experiencing the benefits. You can practice MFR anytime.

Upper Back

Target: upper-back muscles (rhomboids, teres major/minor, latissimus dorsi)

1 Sit on the floor with your knees bent and the foam roller placed behind you about 2 to 3 feet. Lie down on the floor with the foam roller placed right below the shoulder blades and the arms crossed over your chest. Keep your head neutral and slowly bring your chin down slightly toward your chest.

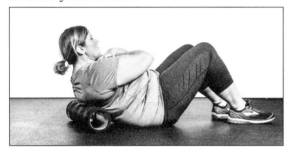

2–3 Lift your butt off the ground by pushing your feet into the floor and pulling your hips up. Now you are in the position to start the myofascial work.

Slowly roll yourself back and forth over the foam roller by using your feet to push your body so that the foam roller hits all areas of your upper- to mid-back (from the base of your neck down across and below your shoulder blades). Keep your arms crossed and be extremely careful not to arch your back over the roller.

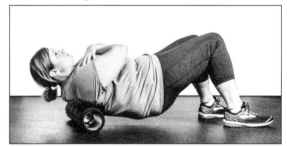

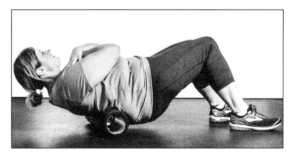

Do 3 to 5 passes and hold any positions that may need additional attention.

Hip Flexors

Target: hip flexors

1 Place both hands in contact with the ground directly under the shoulders and in front of the foam roller. Kneel on your left knee and fully extend your right leg.

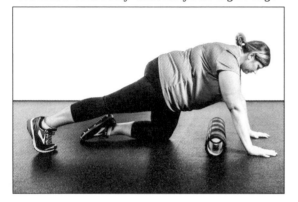

2 Lower down so the foam roller comes in contact with the front of your right upper thigh. Allow the weight of your body to sink into the foam roller. Position your arms so that your right elbow is on the floor; this will keep the low back neutral and prevent a hyperextension. Now use your arms to slowly roll back and forth over the upper thigh/hip flexor. Do 3 to 5 passes and hold any positions that may need additional attention.

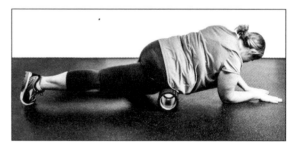

Repeat on the opposite side.

NOTE: In order to isolate the hip flexor, bring the bent knee up and slightly out and in contact with the floor while leaning more body weight on the hip flexor of the extended leg. This will put more body weight pressure on the area you're trying to roll out.

Thighs

Target: quadriceps

1 Get on your hands and knees in a tabletop position with the foam roller directly in front of your knees.

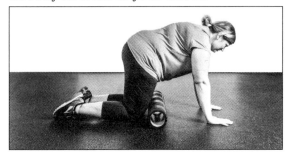

2 Lower down into a plank position so that the foam roller comes in contact with the front of your thighs. Allow the weight of your body to sink into the foam roller. Position your arms so that your elbows are on the floor; this will keep the low back neutral and prevent a hyperextension in the low back. Now use your arms to slowly roll back and forth over your quadriceps (the meaty part of your thighs). Do 3 to 5 passes and hold any positions that may need additional attention.

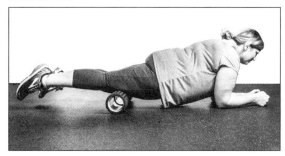

NOTE: If you want to isolate more pressure on one thigh versus the other, shift and lean your body weight more to one side and roll; then switch to the opposite side.

Adductors

Target: adductors

The Position: Lie face-down with the foam roller placed diagonally and underneath your right inner thigh. Bring your knee up and bent over the roller, almost as if you're half straddling the foam roller while lying face down on the ground. Yes, this may feel a little awkward, but it is important to release tight adductors (inner thigh) as it will increase the mobility in your hips.

Position your arms so that you are on your elbows and use the arms to slowly roll back and forth over the adductor muscles. Do 3 to 5 passes and hold any positions that may need additional attention.

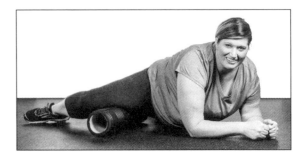

Repeat on the opposite side.

Abductors

Target: abductors and iliotibial (IT) band

The Position: Lie on your left side with the foam roller underneath the hip abductors (upper portion of your leg below the hip bone). Cross your right leg over the left leg and place the left elbow on the floor so that most of your weight is being supported by your right leg and left arm.

Use your arms and legs to slowly roll back and forth for 3 to 5 passes over the left hip abductors.

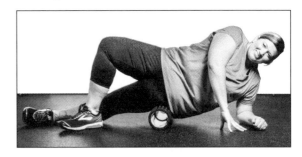

Repeat on the opposite side.

Upper Back on Wall

Target: upper back muscles (rhomboids, teres major/minor, latissimus dorsi)

The Position: Stand 1 to 2 feet away from a wall and place the MFR ball in the upper left back. Lean into the ball so that the ball is pinned between the wall and your upper back, right above the shoulder blade.

While continuing to lean against the ball; slowly move your upper body while keeping the ball in contact with both the wall and your upper back. This movement can be accomplished by moving the upper body from side to side, or by moving the whole body up and down by bending the knees and standing back up.

As you make these movements, the ball will roll across your upper back muscles until you feel it hit a tender/trigger point area. Continue a combined rolling and holding of the ball technique across all affected areas.

Repeat on the opposite side.

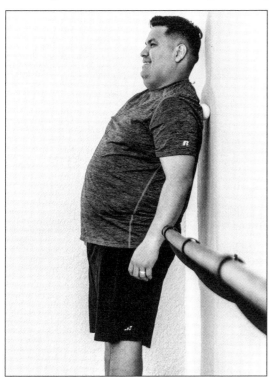

Lower Back

Target: low back muscles (erector spinae)

1 Stand 1 to 2 feet away from a wall and place the MFR ball in the lower left back, just to the right of the spine (or in the meaty area of the low back, called the erector spinae muscles. Lean into the ball so that the ball is pinned between the wall and your lower back.

2 While continuing to lean against the ball, slowly bend the knees and stand back up, allowing the ball to roll up and down the lower back muscles until you feel it hit a tender/trigger point area. Continue a combined rolling and holding technique across all affected areas.

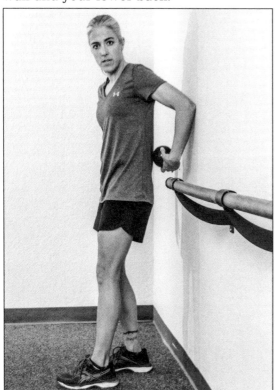

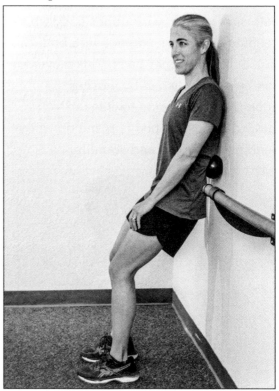

Repeat on the opposite side.

Shoulders

Target: deltoids

1 Stand 1 to 2 feet away from and perpendicular to a wall. Place the MFR ball in the left shoulder (the upper meaty area of the arm, or the deltoid muscle). Lean against the wall so that the ball is in contact with both the wall and your left shoulder.

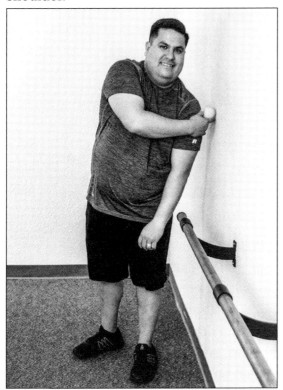

2 While continuing to lean against the ball, slowly roll the ball by bending your knees and standing up again, using your lower body and upper body so that the ball moves into a circular motion against the shoulder muscles. Continue until you feel it hit a tender/trigger point area and then use a combined rolling and holding technique across all affected areas.

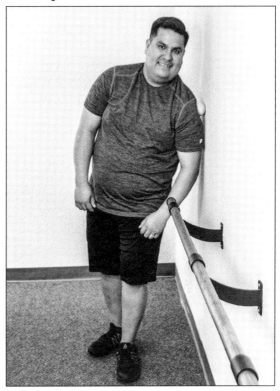

Repeat on the opposite side.

Glutes

Target: butt muscles (gluteus maximus and minimus)

1 Sit on the floor with your right knee bent and right foot flat on the floor and your left leg outstretched and in contact with the floor. Place the MFR ball under the right glute.

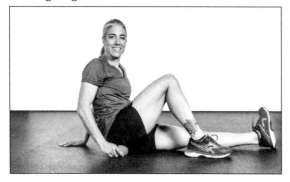

2 Bring your hands behind you for support. Now slowly roll on the ball using your left foot and arms behind you to move your body around on the ball. Do this until you feel the ball hit a tender/trigger point area. Continue a combined rolling and holding technique across all affected areas.

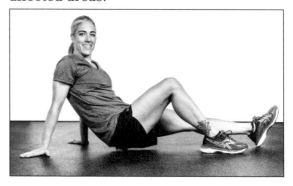

Repeat on the opposite side.

NOTE: If you are unable to get onto the floor, you can sit in a chair and then place the ball under your right glute. Once the ball is positioned, shift your hips side to side to apply pressure in the glute muscles; reposition the ball and repeat. Repeat on the opposite side.

Calves

Target: calf muscles (gastrocnemius and soleus)

1 Sit on the floor with your left knee bent and left foot flat on the floor and your right leg outstretched and in contact with the floor. Place the MFR ball under the right calf.

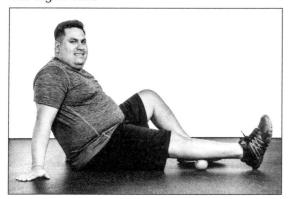

2 Bring your hands behind you for support. Use your hands and your left foot to lift your butt up off the ground and simultaneously roll the ball forward and back over the calf muscle until you feel the ball hit a tender/trigger point area. To target all affected areas, you'll need to rotate your right foot and allow the ball to roll across the lateral (outside) and medial (inside) areas of the calf muscle. Continue a combined rolling and holding technique across all affected areas.

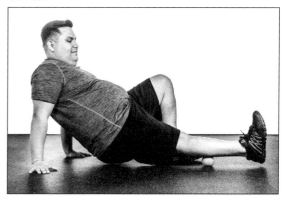

Repeat on the opposite side.

Feet

The Position: From a seated position, place the MFR ball under the middle portion or arch of your left bare foot. Roll the foot back and forth for 3 to 5 passes. Use a combined rolling and holding technique across all affected areas.

NOTE: To add a little pressure to the roll on the foot, you can either lean on the knees while rolling, or do this exercise standing.

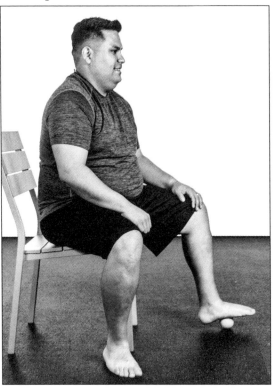

Repeat on the opposite side.

Chapter 4

CARDIO FOR WEIGHT LOSS

Cardiovascular/aerobic exercise involves moving large muscle groups in a rhythmic motion for an extended period of time. Essentially, exercise that involves continuous repetitive motion is cardio, such as walking, bicycling, swimming, rowing, jogging, or taking an aerobics class. Cardio is the principal form of exercise for burning fat calories, and there is a science behind exercising for weight loss. Of course, cardio is also important for improved heart health, and improving your cardiovascular health must be one of your goals, because without a healthy heart, your weight-loss endeavor may be cut short.

No matter where you are in your weight-loss journey, cardio should always be a part of your fitness regimen. Even post-weight-loss surgery, your medical team will get you up and moving the same day of your procedure. This helps the healing process and prevents the risk of blood clots. You'll be asked to start walking the day of or within the first day of surgery and to gradually increase the frequency and duration of your walks each week.

The only real exception here is if your excess weight restricts you from being able to perform traditional cardiovascular exercise. Two examples are if you are physically unable to do cardio (such as walking) because it causes too much pain on the joints or your deconditioned state prevents you from being able to get up and do it. If this is the case, start with the mobility routines outlined previously or try the "Seated Exercise" routine I've outlined in this chapter. As you lose weight, it will become easier to move and you'll be able to do more regimented cardio workouts.

UNDERSTANDING YOUR ZONES

Now the only way to know exactly where your body burns fat most efficiently is to do metabolic testing—specifically, a VO2 max assessment. Check your local area to see if there are any companies that offer this type of testing. You can also search the KORR website (korr.com/facility-finder) to find if a facility offers this testing near you.

A VO2 max assessment can pinpoint the heart rate, or intensity, at which you burn the most fat. It can also determine when you burn 50 percent carbs and 50 percent fat, something called your aerobic base, as well as your threshold point, or the heart rate at which you begin to burn 100 percent carbohydrates. What's cool about this test is that it is independent of any blood pressure medications you might be taking; so, whatever the test results reveal, these are the heart rate zones that will be individualized based on how you metabolize calories during exercise.

If you are on blood pressure medications (specifically a beta blocker) and your doctor changes your medication, you will need to get retested as your zones could change. Your zones will also change as you become more fit, so I recommend you get retested every three to four months as long as you're progressing with your heart rate training.

To make this relatively simple to understand, I'm going to outline four different heart rate zones. You'll determine these zones either via the test results of a VO2 max assessment or by using a Rating of Perceived Exertion (RPE) scale. If you're able to get the metabolic testing done, make sure you ask your fitness professional the following three questions concerning the test results:

1) At what heart rate did you burn the greatest percentage of fat? This is the heart rate when you're utilizing the most oxygen; if you're a good fat burner you'll actually burn 100 percent fat at this heart rate. Physiologically, you burn 100 percent fat when your Respiratory Exchange Ratio (RER) is 0.70. This value can be extrapolated from the VO2 max assessment.

2) At what heart rate did you start burning 100 percent carbohydrates? This is the heart rate when you're no longer utilizing oxygen to burn calories, and thus, you're anaerobic (without oxygen). Physiologically, you burn 100 percent carbohydrates when your RER is 1.00. This means that you expired just as much carbon-dioxide as oxygen you took in.

3) What was your max heart rate? This is the heart rate when you maxed out or when you reached your VO2 max. Physiologically, you achieve a max VO2 when you hit an RER of 1.1; this is the definition of true VO2 max. However, depending on your fitness level you might not be able to physically hit 1.1 on the RER. It's okay if you don't; you'll simply use the heart rate when your rating of perceived exertion was 10 instead. That is still your max and should have occurred when you hit your highest VO2 value.

If you know these three heart rates, you'll be able to determine your zones. The health and fitness professional that performs your assessment should be able to give you your zones, or at a minimum tell you these three heart rates: max fat burn, max carb burn, and max heart rate. If the health and fitness professional gives you training zones, simply double check that the zones they set up for you coincide with these heart rate values detailed below.

If you can't get the testing done, use the Rating of Perceived Exertion (RPE) scale to determine your zones. Below is a modified RPE scale; be sure to note the descriptions correlated with the numbers in the chart.

Rating of Perceived Exertion (RPE) Scale

RPE	DESCRIPTION
0	Nothing at All
0.5	Just Noticeable
1	Very Light
2	Light
3	Moderate
4	Somewhat Hard
5–6	Hard
7–9	Very Hard
10	Very, Very Hard

RPE = 0	This is how you feel prior to starting any exercise—no exertion.
RPE = 3–4	You should be able to maintain a conversation with minimal effort.
RPE = 5–6	You should still be able to talk, but it will be difficult to speak in full sentences.
RPE = 7–8	Very difficult to speak more than a few words at a time.
RPE = 10	Max exertion; intensity you can't maintain for more than 1 minute.

DETERMINING YOUR ZONES

Now that you either have your VO2 numbers or have reviewed the RPE scale, you can determine your cardio training zones. Use the explanations below to figure out your personal training zones.

Fat Burning Zone (FBZ): This is a low to moderate intensity at which you'll be able to carry on a conversation with ease while exercising. It's also the intensity at which you burn the greatest percentage of fat. If you're just starting an exercise program or have weight loss as your primary objective, you should spend 50 percent or more of your time each week exercising in this zone.

Use the heart rate at Max Fat Burn from your VO2 assessment and create a 10 to 20 beat zone around that value. This will be your FBZ. So, if your Max Fat Burn occurred at a heart rate of 90 beats per minute, your FBZ may be 85 to 95, 85 to 100, or 85 to 105 beats per minute (BPM). If you're using the RPE scale, your FBZ will be the intensity from 1 to 4 on the scale.

Fit Zone (FZ): This is a moderate intensity at which you'd be able to exercise for an extended period of time. You're able to talk, but will need to catch your breath occasionally and it will be difficult to speak in full sentences. You'll generally burn about 50 percent carbs and 50 percent fat calories when exercising in this zone.

Create your Fit Zone by adding 10 to 20 beats from the largest value of your FBZ. This will be your FZ. Using the example above, if your FBZ was 85 to 100, then your FZ may be 100 to 110, 100 to 115 or 100 to 120 BPM. If you're using the RPE scale, your FZ will be the intensity from 5 to 6 on the scale.

Threshold Zone (TZ): This is a high intensity at which you will generally only be able to exercise for short bursts of time (1 to 15 minutes). It is also where you'll be burning 100 percent carbohydrates and make the greatest impact for improving your heart health. If your main objective is to improve your heart health, you'll want to incorporate this level of intensity into your weekly routine.

Use the heart rate at Max Carb Burn from your VO2 assessment and create a 10 to 20 beat zone around that value. This will be your TZ. So, if your Max Carb Burn occurred at a heart rate of 145 beats per minute, your TZ may be 135 to 145, 135 to 150 or 135 to 155 BPM.

NOTE: Your TZ should never exceed your Max Heart Rate value. If it does, you'll need to readjust your previous zones to make sure this zone doesn't go over the Max HR. If you're using the RPE scale, your TZ will be the intensity from 7 to 8 on the scale.

Red Zone (RZ): This is a very high intensity at which you may or may not be able to exercise. This zone is for the more fit person, but it does a lot to improve cardiovascular fitness, i.e, "heart health"! Keep in mind that you'll be burning all carbohydrates in this zone, so it's not necessary or conducive to train here if your primary goal is weight loss.

Create your Red Zone by adding 10 to 20 beats from your largest value of your TZ. This will be your RZ. Using the example above, if your TZ was 135 to 145, then your RZ may be 145 to 155, 145 to 160 or 145 to 165 BPM.

NOTE: Like the TZ, your RZ should never go over your Max Heart Rate value. If it does, you'll need to readjust your previous zones to make sure this zone doesn't go over the Max HR. If you're using the RPE scale, your RZ will be the intensity from 9 to 10 on the scale.

If your primary objective is weight loss, you'll want to spend most of your time exercising in the fat burning and fit zones. If you're looking to improve heart health, you'll need to spend time exercising in your threshold or red zones. As you increase your overall fitness and get closer to your ideal weight, you'll ultimately want to do some cardio in all different zones throughout the week. This style of training will be most beneficial in creating an efficient fat-burning machine and improving your heart health.

TRACKING YOUR HEART RATE

Regardless of whether you're using heart rate or RPE to monitor your intensity during your workouts, invest in a good heart rate monitor (HRM). An HRM is a personal monitoring device that tracks your heart rate in real time. I personally prefer HRMs that come with both the transmitter chest strap and the receiver wrist display. I've found these to be the most accurate as they are tracking your heart rate at the heart versus a pulse rate at the wrist, which can be several beats off. Many models today contain a Bluetooth feature that can connect the HRM to your smartwatch or smartphone. I've become partial to Polar HRMs—Polar was the first company to introduce a wearable heart rate monitoring device in 1978. Ideally, I want you to wear an HRM even if you're using RPE to track intensity because over time you'll know the heart rate that correlates with your RPE (e.g., when you're at an RPE of 3 to 4, you'll know that your heart rate is generally between 110 and 120 BPM).

CARDIO WORKOUTS WITH PROGRESSIONS

All the workouts outlined in this chapter are designed to be cardiovascular. Other than the Seated Exercise Routine, I did not specify what type of cardio to do. Walking, biking, swimming, hiking, and other types of activities are examples of modalities of exercise. You should choose the modality that is best for you based on your medical conditions, fitness level, what is available to you, and what you enjoy doing. I'm most concerned about your intensity of the cardio—the heart rate you achieve—rather than what type of cardio you perform.

SEATED EXERCISE ROUTINE

This non-traditional cardio program is designed for the person who has too much joint pain to perform traditional cardiovascular exercise (such as walking), is too deconditioned to physically get up and do cardio, or simply doesn't have the right equipment accessible to them. The beauty of this routine is that anyone can do these exercises anywhere because all you need is your own body. It can even be a great office workout if you spend a lot of time sitting at your desk for work. You can still monitor your intensity as you perform this routine, either by tracking your heart rate or using the RPE scale.

Perform 5 to 30 repetitions (start with 5 and build up to 30) for each exercise, move directly from one exercise to the next (ideally without resting; work up to this), and continue for the full workout.

Once you've done each exercise for the specified number of repetitions, continue through the circuit a second, third, or fourth time. Start with 5 minutes total duration of exercise and build up to 30 or more minutes.

Forward Punch

Target: chest/shoulders

1 Bring both arms up with fists clasped and positioned in front of your chest with elbows down.

2 Slowly extend the right arm out in front until it is almost to full extension, rotating your wrist inward so the palm faces down with knuckles up. Do not lock out the elbow.

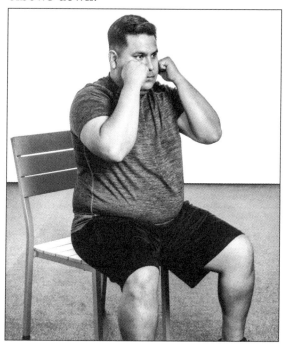

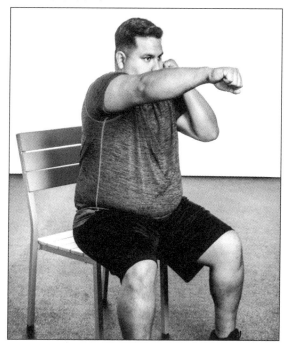

Return to starting position, switch sides, and repeat.

Continue alternating for 5 to 30 repetitions on each side.

March in Place (Seated)

Target: legs

1 Sit up tall on the front half of a chair with feet shoulder-width apart and flat on the floor. Lifting your right foot off the ground, slowly bring the right leg straight up. Lift the foot as far off the ground as is comfortable for you.

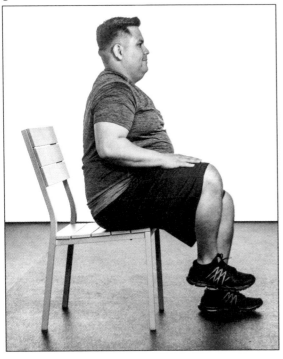

2 Return to starting position, switch sides, and repeat.

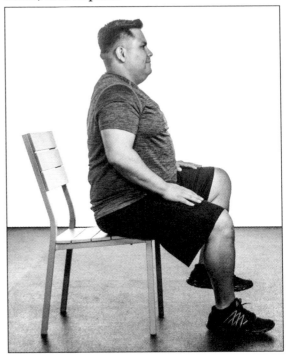

Continue alternating in a "marching" pattern for 5 to 30 repetitions on each side.

Overhead Punch

Target: shoulders

1 Sit up tall on the front half of a chair with feet shoulder-width apart and flat on the floor. Bring both arms up with fists clasped and positioned in front of your chest with elbows down.

2 Slowly extend your right arm straight up overhead until the arm is almost to a full extension and the palm is facing in toward the center of your body. Do not lock out the elbow.

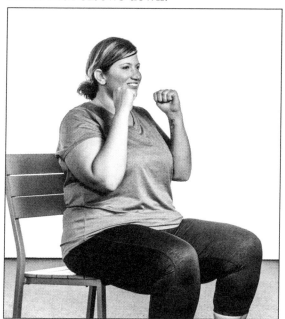

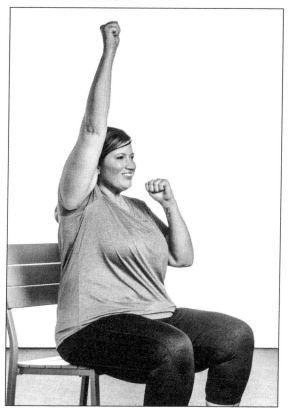

Return to starting position, switch sides, and repeat.

Continue alternating for 5 to 30 repetitions on each side.

Alternating Leg Extension

Target: thighs/quadriceps

1 Sit up tall on the front half of a chair with feet shoulder-width apart and flat on the floor. With your foot flexed, slowly lift the right foot so that the leg is fully extended out in front.

2 Return to starting position, switch sides, and repeat.

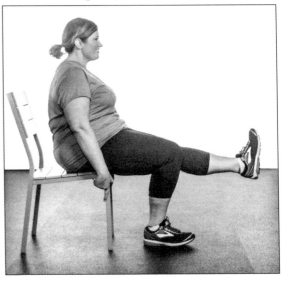

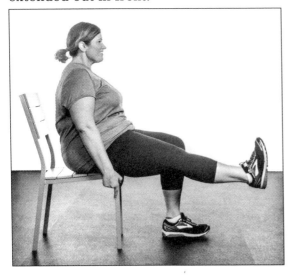

Continue alternating for 5 to 30 repetitions on each side.

Overhead Clap Seated

Target: arms/shoulders

1 Sit up tall on the front half of a chair with feet shoulder-width apart and flat on the floor. Extend both arms out to the sides until parallel to the ground and your palms facing up.

2 Bring both arms up and together until the palms touch or "clap" overhead.

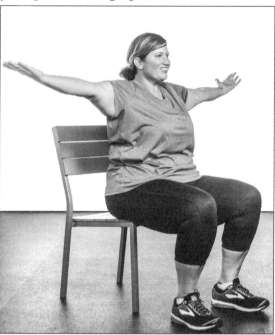

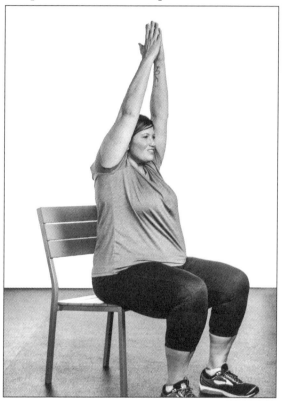

Return to starting position, and continue for 5 to 30 repetitions.

HEART RATE TRAINING

There are countless ways to design a heart rate training program. The heart rate programs described here are great to help get you started. Reference the training zones on page 86 to understand how each zone impacts your overall fitness. Here are the abbreviations again:

Fat Burning Zone (FZ)   Threshold Zone (TZ)

Fit Zone (FZ)   Red Zone (RZ)

Remember to always warm up before starting these workouts. You can use the Range of Motion routine (page 29), or simply do 5 to 10 minutes of a slow/low-intensity exercise to warm up. You'll always want to warm up the muscles you're about to use. So, if you're going to walk, do a slow-paced walk for 5 to 10 minutes as your warm-up and then get into the outlined heart rate zone workout).

Once you've done these different programs for six to eight weeks), you can start coming up with your own heart rate training programs by changing up different components of your workout. I've outlined a few methods of doing so here:

1) Mix up the modality (i.e., the type of cardio exercise equipment you are training on). So if you've been walking for most of your workouts, try cycling, swimming, or doing the elliptical trainer.

2) Change up the duration you spend in the different zones.

3) Increase or decrease the total duration of the workout.

4) Add another zone to your weekly routine (if you've only been working in the Fat Burning and Fit Zones, try doing a workout with part of your time in the Threshold Zone).

Eventually you want to progress to the point where you're doing one to two of each workout every week. In other words, you'd do one or two Max Fat Burning (low intensity), one or two Fit (moderately intense), and one or two Threshold (high intensity) workouts each week. Your body will react to how you train, so the more heart rate zones you end up training in each week, the better your body will burn fat at higher intensities and longer durations. This style of training also builds up your overall cardiovascular fitness so that you're burning more fat calories all the time, even when you're not exercising.

The key is to continue to monitor your heart rate while training, and again, if fat loss is your number one goal, spend approximately 50 to 75 percent of your cardiovascular training in the Fat Burning and Fit Zones. If you've achieved your goal weight and/ or need to improve your heart health, spend approximately 50 to 75 percent of your cardiovascular training in your Fit, Threshold, and Red Zones combined.

Heart Training Programs

	MAX FAT BURNING	FIT TRAINING	THRESHOLD TRAINING
	intensity: low to moderate	intensity: moderate	intensity: high
	target: fat-burning	target: improve fat burning and aerobic fitness	target: improved heart health
WORKOUT 1	5:00 to 60:00 all FBZ *Start with 5 minutes in the Fat Burning Zone and build up your duration until you can do 60 total minutes.*	5:00 to 60:00 all FZ *Start with 5 minutes in the Fit Zone and build up your duration until you can do 60 total minutes.*	45:00 pyramid: • 5:00 FBZ • 5:00 FZ • 10:00 TZ • 5:00 RZ • 10:00 TZ • 5:00 FZ • 5:00 FBZ *You can make this workout longer and more intense by adding time in each zone interval (e.g., 10:00 FBZ, 10:00 FZ, 15:00 TZ, 10:00 RZ, 15:00 TZ, 10:00 FZ, 10:00 FBZ).*
WORKOUT 2	10:00 to 60:00 half/half 5:00 to 30:00 all FBZ 5:00 to 30:00 all FZ *Start with 5 minutes in the FBZ and then 5 minutes in the FZ. Build up your duration until you can do 30 continuous minutes in the FBZ and 30 continuous minutes in the FZ.*	35-minute pyramid 5:00 FBZ 10:00 FZ 5:00 TZ 10:00 FZ 5:00 FBZ *You can make this workout longer and more intense by adding time in each zone interval (e.g., 10:00 FBZ, 15:00 FZ, 10:00 TZ, 15:00 FZ, 10:00 FBZ).*	10:00 to 50:00 intervals • 5:00 FZ • 3:00 TZ • 2:00 RZ *Work within these zones and then cycle back around so that you're doing an interval circuit between the three zones. Complete 2 to 5 circuits.* *Start with 10 minutes and build up your duration until you can do 50 total minutes.*

Heart Training Programs

	MAX FAT BURNING	FIT TRAINING	THRESHOLD TRAINING
	intensity: low to moderate	intensity: moderate	intensity: high
	target: fat-burning	target: improve fat burning and aerobic fitness	target: improved heart health
WORKOUT 3	10:00 to 60:00 of intervals 5:00 FBZ 5:00 FZ Alternate back and forth between these two zones. *Start with 10 minutes and build up your duration until you can do 60 total minutes.*	20:00 staircase 10:00 FBZ 5:00 FZ 5:00 TZ *You can make this workout longer and more intense by adding time in each zone interval or by repeating the staircase.*	40:00 to 60:00 staircase • 10:00 to 15:00 FBZ • 10:00 to 15:00 FZ • 10:00 to 15:00 TZ • 10:00 to 15:00 RZ

5K CHALLENGE

A 5K race would be a great way to bring an added challenge to your workout routine. And you don't have to run the distance; most races today allow walkers to compete, so think about it from a distance standpoint rather than a race or speed challenge. Find an event in your area that is about two to three months away, and then start following one of the training plans below to help get you ready for the event.

Unlike the heart rate training programs outlined in this chapter, when you start training for a distance event, distance will be the main training variable rather than heart rate. However, it is still important to be mindful of your heart rate during training sessions.

Here are some good websites and apps to help you find a race:

Websites:
www.active.com
www.runnersworld.com
www.runningintheusa.com
www.localraces.com

Apps:
Race Finder
ACTIVE
Run America

This six-week training plan is designed to get you ready to walk, jog, or run a 5K race. If you are training to walk rather than jog or run the event, substitute the jog/run training with a fast power walk. I have included strength-training workouts throughout this plan. You can use one of the strength-training programs in Chapter 5 for these workouts. "TB" stands for total body, meaning you'll be working your entire body with these strength workouts. When it lists "cross training" in the plan, this means that I want you to do a different cardio activity than walking, jogging, or running that day. Cycling, rowing, the elliptical trainer, Zumba, cross-country skiing, or swimming are great options. You do not have to perform each workout on the specified day; just be sure to get them all in for the week.

	MON	TUE	WED	THU	FRI	SAT	SUN
WEEK 1	30:00 cross training	1-mile run	TB Strength Train	1.5-mile interval (¼ mile fast run/ walk and 2:00 recovery slow walk x 6)	TB Strength Train	REST	30:00 walk/jog (4:00/1:00 splits)
WEEK 2	40:00 cross training	1.5-mile run	TB Strength Train	2-mile interval (¼ mile fast run/walk and 2:00 recovery slow walk x 8)	TB Strength Train	REST	40:00 walk/jog (3:00/2:00 splits)
WEEK 3	40:00 cross training	2-mile run	TB Strength Train	2.5-mile interval (¼ mile fast run/ walk and 2:00 recovery slow walk x 10)	TB Strength Train	REST	45:00 walk/jog (2:00/3:00 splits)
WEEK 4	45:00 cross training	2.5-mile run	TB Strength Train	2.5-mile interval (¼ mile fast run/ walk and 2:00 recovery slow walk x 10)	TB Strength Train	REST	45:00 walk/jog (1:00/4:00 splits)
WEEK 5	45:00 cross training	3-mile run	TB Strength Train	2.75-mile interval (¼ mile fast run/ walk and 2:00 recovery slow walk x 11)	TB Strength Train	REST	50:00 power walk or run the whole time
WEEK 6	20:00 cross training	2-mile run	TB Strength Train	1.5-mile walk	REST	1-mile run or walk	5K RACE DAY

TRIATHLON "SPRINT DISTANCE" TRAINING PLAN

Maybe you're looking for a bigger challenge—triathlon may be calling your name. Triathlons combine swimming, biking, and running into one event. There are several different triathlon distances (such as sprint, Olympic, and Ironman) to accommodate varying skill and fitness levels, but you can start with what's called a "sprint distance" and build from there. Sprint distances may vary from race to race.

A sprint distance triathlon typically equates to a 0.5-mile (750-meter) swim, 12.4-mile (20-kilometer) bike ride, and 3.1-mile (5-kilometer) run. This training plan will include swim distances in meters (m) and the bike or run distances in time in minutes or distance in miles. A typical pool is either 25m or 50m (Olympic size) in length. You can do your run training on a treadmill, but be sure to spend at least one of the training runs throughout the week on pavement to condition your body for the harder surface.

I've also included one practice training where you'll be doing all three activities so that you can become familiar with the transitioning component of this race. Transitioning is the time between exercise modalities in the triathlon (i.e., the time between finishing your swim and starting the bike and the time between finishing the bike and beginning the run). If your actual race is going to have an open-water swim (i.e., a lake or an ocean), be sure to do a few of your swim trainings in that type of water. I also have strength-training workouts throughout this training plan. You can use one of the strength training programs in Chapter 5 for these workouts. You'll also see "brick" listed in the training plan. A brick triathlon workout is where you go from one discipline of exercise straight into another, typically bike to run. "TB" stands for total body, meaning you'll be working your entire body with these strength workouts.

Here's your 10-week Sprint Tri training program:

	MON	TUE	WED	THU	FRI	SAT	SUN
WEEK 1	OFF	400m swim	45:00 bike	20:00 run	OFF	TB Strength Workout (2 sets x 12 reps)	OFF
WEEK 2	OFF	600m swim	45:00 bike	30:00 run	OFF	TB Strength Workout (2 sets x 12 reps)	Brick 60:00 bike 15:00 run
WEEK 3	OFF	800m swim	OFF	2-mile run	OFF	TB Strength Workout (2 sets x 12 reps)	Brick 45:00 bike 20:00 run
WEEK 4	OFF	1000m swim	45:00 bike	3-mile run	OFF	TB Strength Workout (2 sets x 12 reps)	Brick 14-mile bike 20:00 run
WEEK 5	OFF	1200m swim	50:00 bike	3.5-mile run	OFF	TB Strength Workout (2 sets x 12 reps)	Brick 14-mile bike 30:00 run
WEEK 6	OFF	1500m swim	60:00 bike	4-mile run	OFF	*If race day is open-water swim, swim in open water today*	OFF
WEEK 7	OFF	800m swim	10-mile bike ride	2-mile run	OFF	Practice Tri • 30:00 swim • 16-mile bike ride • 3-mile run TB Strength Workout (2 sets x 12 reps)	OFF
WEEK 8	OFF	1500m swim	50:00 bike	4-mile run	OFF	Brick • 18-mile bike • 3-mile run	Open-Water Swim 20:00 okay to combine this workout with previous day's workout

	MON	TUE	WED	THU	FRI	SAT	SUN
WEEK 9	OFF	800m swim	10-mile bike	2-mile run	OFF	TB Strength Workout (2 sets x 12 reps)	OFF
WEEK 10	OFF	800m swim	45:00 bike	2-mile run	OFF	Walk 1 to 2 miles	SPRINT DISTANCE TRIATHLON

Once you complete a race, chances are high that you'll be inspired to sign up for another. I only outlined a few training plans for a handful of race types. There are many more race types you could sign up for, such as different bike distances, adventure races, Spartan races, duathlons (run, bike, run), and more. These different races can be incredible motivators to keep you consistent with your exercise. If you want to look for a new event to participate in, simply search Google for the type of race you're interested in.

Chapter 5

STRENGTH TRAINING FOR WEIGHT LOSS

Strength or resistance training is often overlooked when trying to lose weight. This is partially due to the fear of gaining weight and in part from a lack of understanding how to properly strength training. First, let's squash the idea that strength training will make you gain weight. If the program is designed properly, you will not gain weight from strength training. In fact, the primary focus of strength training is to preserve the lean muscle mass through the weight-loss phase. Strength training will help change your body composition by decreasing fat and maintaining or increasing a little bit of lean muscle. This will ultimately keep or increase your metabolic rate, which determines how well you burn fat and total calories. In fact, strength training is an important component to any weight-loss program. In addition to weight management, strength training improves your posture and balance, prevents injury, increases bone density, decreases joint pain, improves strength, prevents disease, and reduces stress.

What kind of strength-training program you choose will largely depend on your workout environment as well as what equipment you have available. Once you've decided where you'll be working out (such as at a gym, at home, or in a park), you can choose a strength routine that will work in that environment. I've outlined two total-body strength programs in this chapter.

SETS AND REPS

"Repetitions," or reps, refers to a complete motion of an exercise. A set is the number of times you perform a group of consecutive reps. For example, if you do 2 sets of 12 reps for a dumbbell biceps curl, that means you'll perform 12 full repetitions of the biceps curl and you'll do those 12 consecutive reps two times. (A dumbbell is a short bar with weights at the end of each side; you can use a single dumbbell or two at a time.)

Since weight loss is your main objective, keep your reps between 12 and 20. This is most conducive for muscle toning and losing body fat without gaining a lot of muscle mass. If your main objective is muscle building and increasing muscular strength, you'd keep your reps between 4 and 10. Reps between 10 to 12 are best for weight maintenance. Choose a weight that will allow you to perform the exercises with proper form yet be challenging on the last 2 or 3 repetitions. Perfect form with a lighter weight is always better than poor form with a heavier weight.

How many sets and reps along with the rest interval and amount of weight for each exercise will depend on your level of fitness and experience with strength training. Determine your starting point based on the descriptions here and set up your routine accordingly (keep in mind that the strength routines in this book are geared toward weight loss). You can increase the intensity of your strength training sessions by modifying the number of sets, reps, rest intervals between these sets/reps, incorporating short cardio-type exercises within the strength workout, or increasing the total number of strength training workouts throughout the week. These different progression methods are explained in greater detail below.

FITNESS LEVELS AND INTENSITY PROGRESSION

BEGINNER

If you haven't exercised in one or more years, have never done strength training, or are extremely deconditioned, perform 1 to 2 sets of each exercise and rest for 1 to 2 minutes after each exercise. Do a strength training workout 1 or 2 times per week and use a routine that is either total body or split into upper body one day and lower body another.

Follow the number of repetitions outlined in each strength program. As you increase your fitness, move onto an intermediate- or advanced-style of strength training.

INTERMEDIATE

If you've been exercising consistently for one month or longer, you'll be ready to perform 2 to 3 sets of each exercise and either circuit or complex/super set each exercise (explanation follows). Do a strength-training workout 2 or 3 times per week and use a routine that is either total-body or split into muscles groups.

Circuit training involves performing multiple exercises in a row with little to no rest between each exercise. You can design a circuit in one of two ways: 1) grouping 3 to 6 exercises together into what I call a "mini-circuit"; or 2) grouping all strength exercises into one "big-circuit." Two to three minutes of rest are taken at the completion of each mini- or big-circuit.

Complexing/Super-setting your exercise involves performing two different exercises back to back with little to no rest between the exercises. Thirty to sixty seconds of rest are taken after each one set of paired exercises. If you are complexing or super-setting your exercises, do not perform exercises using the same muscle groups consecutively (e.g., chest press followed by a pec fly; both target the chest/pectoral muscles). This is a pre-exhaustive style of strength training that can cause hypertrophy (increasing the muscle size) and is not recommend for weight loss unless you are trying to build muscle or break out of a plateau.

ADVANCED

If you've been exercising for six or more months, perform 3 to 5 sets of each exercise. Use a combination of circuits, complexing/super-setting, pyramid, drop sets, high volume, or high-intensity interval training (HIIT). Circuit and complexing/super-setting were explained previously; descriptions for the latter four are outlined here.

Pyramid style of strength training deals with manipulating the number of reps into a pyramid. For example, you could do 3 sets of 12-15-12 reps or 5 sets of 12-15-20-15-12 for example. Combine this style of training with either a mini- or big-circuit.

Drop sets are like a pyramid method, but instead of going from a lower number of sets to higher and back down, you'd simply start out high and drop the number of reps with each set. For example, do 3 sets of 20, 16, and 12 reps. You can also do drop sets with timed intervals; for example, do 3 sets of 60, 45, and 30 seconds timed reps.

High volume is just that: a high number of sets and reps. Timed intervals work well to satisfy this progression, especially when combined with circuit training, pyramid, or drop sets. You'll want to keep your reps high (i.e., closer to the 20-rep mark), and you may even go over 20 reps when doing timed intervals for, say, 90, 60, or 45 seconds.

HIIT training brings cardio into the mix of strength training, and these cardio bouts will increase the intensity of the strength routine. This method is best used when combined with either circuit or complexing/super-setting your routine. For example, you could add 30 to 60 seconds of moderately high-intensity cardio—like jumping jacks, running, rowing, or boxing—between each mini-circuit or pair of exercises in a superset. This style of strength training will give you a higher total calorie burn and adds an aerobic benefit to your strength-training workout (which is generally anaerobic in nature).

If you have a restriction or limitation, avoid movements that may complicate that condition. If you are not sure which movements will complicate your restriction or limitation, keep in mind that joint pain is never healthy pain. If you experience joint pain, modify that exercise or avoid it all together. You can always substitute one of the other exercises in this chapter or create a modified movement that will not aggravate your limitation.

Now you have a good baseline for why strength training is important for weight loss and understand the different strength-training levels and methods for progression. I will only be outlining the exercises within each program. The order of how you perform the exercises within each program, along with how many sets, reps, and the rest interval in between will depend on your fitness level and which level of progression (page 102) you decide to use.

You can do total body 2 or 3 times per week, split upper body and lower body 2 to 4 times per week, or break it down into muscle-group strength workouts throughout the week (i.e., back and biceps, chest and triceps, etc.).

The programs here are total-body workouts, but if you'd rather do muscle splits, please read through the Muscle Splits Programs (page 129) to understand how to set up this type of strength program. It is important to leave one whole day of rest between strength training muscle groups. In other words, if you do a total-body strength workout on Tuesday, don't do it again until Thursday or Friday. Leave Wednesday as a recovery day from strength. You can do cardio back to back, but if you're strength training, don't train the same muscle group on consecutive days.

TOTAL BODY STRENGTH PROGRAM 1

This routine is designed to be accomplished in the comforts of your own home or at a gym or other fitness facility. You will need dumbbells and a bench.

Chair Squat

Target: legs; hamstrings, quadriceps, glutes

1 Stand tall about 1 inch from a bench or chair with your feet hip-width apart, your arms at your sides, and your back to the chair. Look straight ahead. Inhale and slowly sit back, bending at the waist and the knees and keeping the back straight. Be sure to sit back into the exercise and do not allow the knees to come too far over the toes (this puts strain on the knee joint rather than using your lower-body muscles).

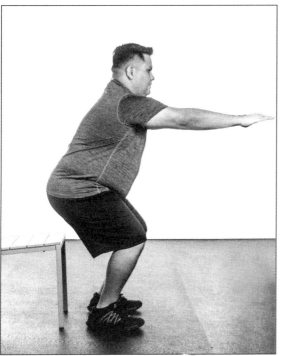

2 Slowly release your weight all the way into the bench or chair.

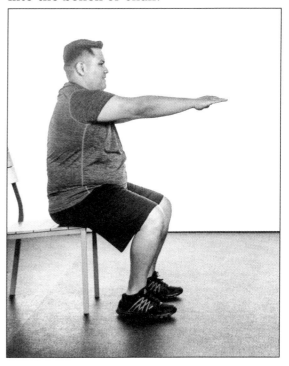

Exhale and stand up to the starting position.

NOTE: Progressing this exercise to make it more challenging would involve barely touching the chair, then not touching the chair at all (i.e., performing a free squat), to using dumbbells (hold a dumbbell in each hand) for added resistance.

Dumbbell Incline Bench Press

Target: chest; pectorals

1 Lie on your back on an incline bench with a dumbbell in each hand and your arms fully extended, but not locked out, in front of your chest with the palms forward.

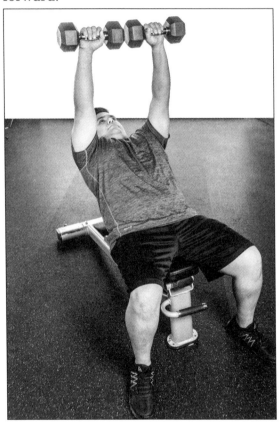

2 Inhale and slowly bring the dumbbells down so that your elbows are bent at 90 degrees.

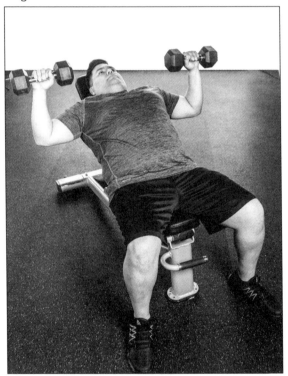

Exhale and slowly push the dumbbells up and back to the starting position.

NOTE: This exercise can also be done using a barbell. I start most overweight to obese people with the incline bench rather a flat bench because it puts less strain on the low back and is often much easier to get in and out. Once you've developed enough strength and/or lost some of your weight, you may prefer to use a flat bench position for this exercise.

Dumbbell Bent-Over Row

Target: back; rhomboids, latissimus dorsi, teres major, teres minor

1 With a dumbbell in each hand, stand tall with your feet shoulder-width apart. Keep your back straight and bend over at the waist, allowing your arms to extend down with the palms facing in. Keep a slight bend in the knees and stick your butt out. Inhale.

2 Exhale and slowly pull both arms up and back, squeezing the shoulder blades together, until the dumbbells are close to your rib cage.

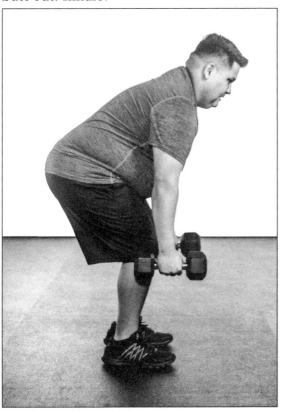

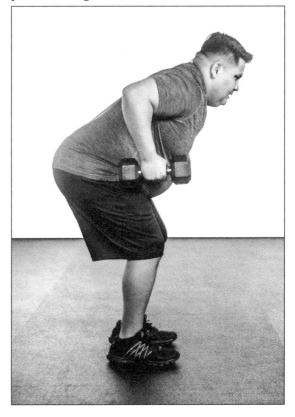

Slowly release your arms back to the starting position. Do not allow your shoulders to roll forward when you get to the final position; keep the shoulders back and down.

Seated Dumbbell Bent-Knee Raise

Target: legs; quadriceps

1 Sit on a bench with feet hip-width apart. Place a single dumbbell on your right thigh, close to the knee, and hold it in place with the right hand. Inhale.

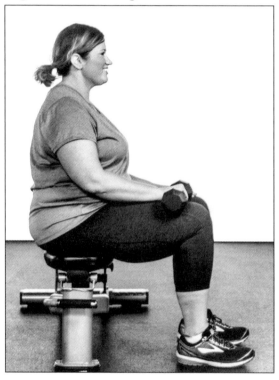

2 Exhale and slowly lift your right leg straight up and take your right foot off the ground. Be sure to keep the back straight and do not rock or lean back during the movement.

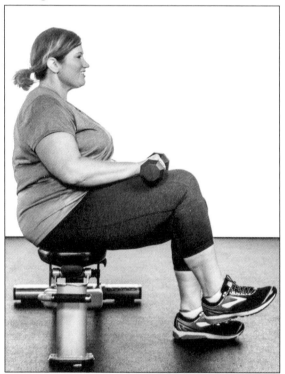

Slowly return the foot to the floor. Continue for the full number of repetitions.

Repeat on the opposite side.

Dumbbell Deadlift

Target: legs/core; hamstrings and low back

1 Stand tall with feet hip-width apart. Grasp a dumbbell in each hand and hold them in front of your thighs with your arms extended.

2 Inhale and slowly bend at the waist while keeping your back straight and maintaining a slight bend in the knees. Continue to bend at the waist until you feel a light stretch/pull in the back of the legs (hamstrings). Keep the dumbbells close to the fronts of your legs.

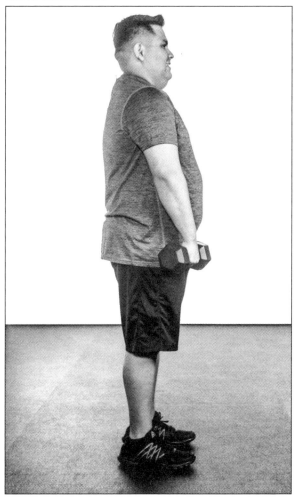

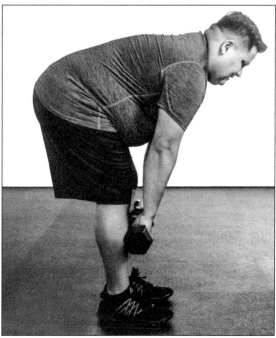

Exhale and lift while maintaining a flat back until you return to your starting position. Be sure to squeeze the glutes (buttocks) at the top of the motion.

Incline Bench Sit-Up

Target: core; abdominals

1 Position the bench at an incline (the greater the incline the easier the sit-up). Lie down on the bench with your arms crossed and in contact with the chest and your chin slightly tucked. Inhale.

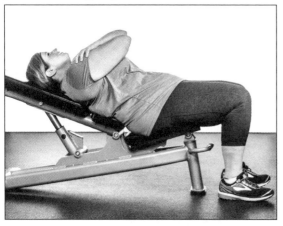

2 Exhale and slowly lift and sit-up off of the bench. Keep your arms in contact with your chest, sit all the way up, and round the back by bringing the elbows toward your thighs.

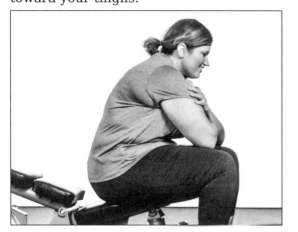

3 Curl your spine and slowly release your body back into the bench, leading with your low back. You want to feel as if you're slowly bringing one vertebrae at a time back in contact with the bench.

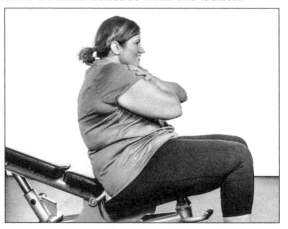

NOTE: As you increase abdominal strength, bring the incline of the bench down until you can perform full sit-ups from the floor.

Dumbbell Front Raise

Target: shoulders; anterior deltoids

1 Grasp a dumbbell in each hand and stand tall with feet hip-width apart and arms extended. Inhale.

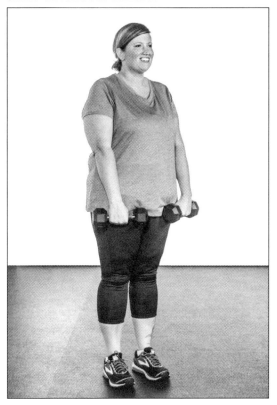

2 Exhale and slowly lift the dumbbells straight out in front of you with ridged arms, but keeping a slight bend in each elbow. Continue to lift until your arms are parallel with the floor.

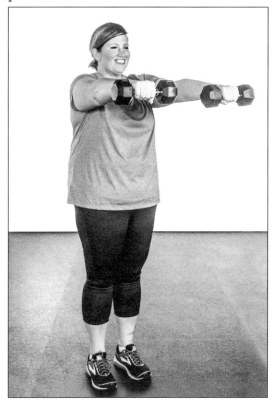

Inhale and slowly lower the dumbbells back to the starting position.

21 Guns

Target: arms; biceps

1 Grasp a dumbbell in each hand and stand tall with arms extended, palms facing forward (supinated), and feet hip-width apart.

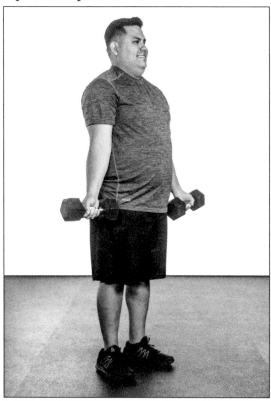

2 Inhale. Exhale and slowly curl the arms up to a 90-degree bend at the elbow.

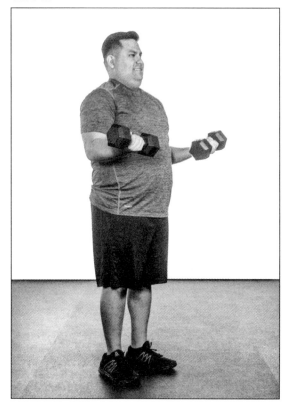

Inhale and return the dumbbells to their starting position. Repeat this halfway-up motion for 7 repetitions.

3 Exhale and curl the dumbbells all the way up to the shoulders.

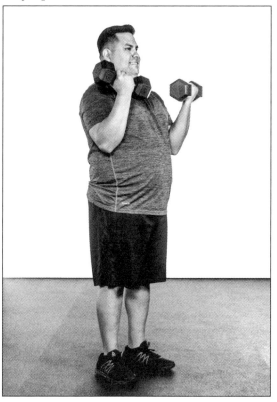

Inhale and lower the dumbbells to a 90-degree bend at the elbow. Repeat this halfway down motion for 7 repetitions.

4 Now you will curl the dumbbells in a complete range of motion. Start with arms fully extended and curl up to your shoulders. Exhale as you lift or curl the weight up to the shoulders and inhale as you lower the weight back down to full extension. Repeat this entire range of motion for 7 repetitions.

NOTE: You will essentially curl the dumbbell weight half way up 7 times, half way down 7 times, and in a full range of motion 7 times for 21 total curls. If you are performing a different number of total repetitions, you'll want to split it up so that you curl one third of the repetitions half way up, one third half way down, and one third in a full range of motion.

Dumbbell Skull Crusher

Target: arms; triceps

1 Lie on your back on an incline bench with a dumbbell in each hand. Extend your arms out in front of your chest with a slight bend in each elbow and palms facing in.

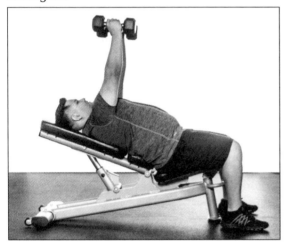

2 Inhale and slowly lower the dumbbells down until they are positioned next to each ear. Keep the elbows high so that they are stacked over your shoulders.

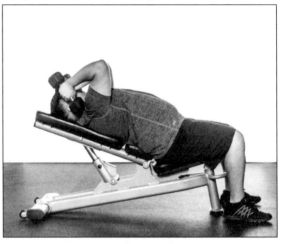

Exhale and push dumbbells up and back to their starting position.

Bridge

Target: legs/core; hamstrings, glutes, low back

1 Lie on your back with knees bent at 90 degrees, feet flat on the floor, and arms flat on the floor with palms facing down. Inhale.

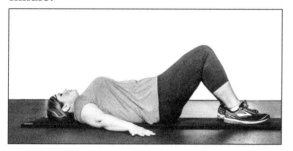

2 Exhale and slowly push the hips up so that your butt rises off the floor and your arms and palms stay in contact with the floor. Hold for one count.

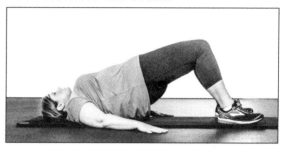

Inhale and return to the starting position.

NOTE: You can progress this exercise, making it more difficult, by holding a dumbbell at your hips or by moving to a single-leg bridge.

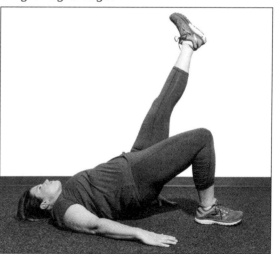

Dumbbell Calf Raise

Target: calves; gastrocneumius, soleus

1 Stand with feet shoulder-width apart and grasp a dumbbell in each hand with arms extended at your sides. Inhale.

2 Exhale and slowly rise onto your toes and hold for one count.

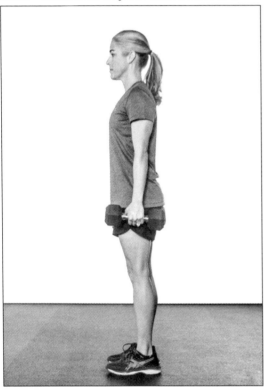

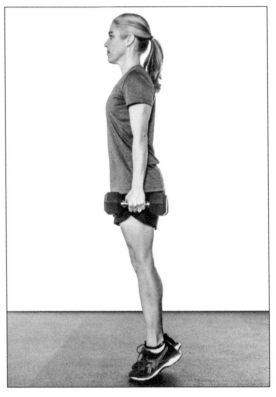

Slowly release and be careful not to rock back onto your heels.

Incline Plank

Target: core; abdominals, obliques, low back

1 Position your elbows on bench shoulder-width apart. Be sure the elbows are stacked directly underneath your shoulders. Step the right foot back with the left foot underneath the hips.

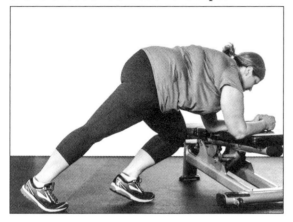

2 Step the left foot back so that your body is in a full plank position (back straight, slight bend in the knees, and butt down). Engage your abdominals, glutes, quadriceps, and low back muscles. Do not let your back sway.

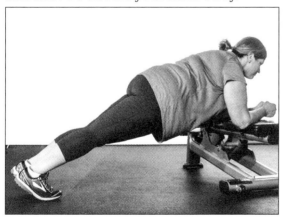

Inhale and exhale in a controlled rhythm while maintaining this plank position for the indicated time (start with a 10-second hold and progress from there).

NOTE: As you increase strength you can increase the duration of time that you hold the plank and then eventually perform this exercise at a lower incline. Ideally, you'll work toward transitioning to a full plank on the floor.

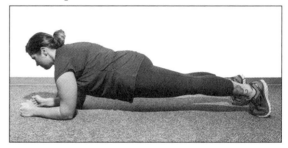

TOTAL BODY STRENGTH PROGRAM 2

This routine is designed to be accomplished anywhere, anytime, which is ideal if you spend a lot of time traveling. You can do this routine in the comforts of your own home or in an office, a hotel room, a gym, or outside.

For some of the exercises in this routine, you will need a resistance band. The resistance band is an easy piece of fitness equipment that you can take anywhere. Throughout the workout I will instruct you to wrap the band around a secure object. Here are three examples of that:

- Hold a resistance band with both hands near the center of the band so that the handles are equal distance apart. Place the center of that band along the narrow side of a door, even with the doorknobs, and then wrap each side of the band around the door knobs.

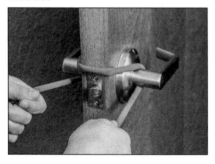

- Loop a resistance band around a secure object while threading one handle through the other and cinching it down until the band is wrapped tightly around the object. Once secure, take the free single handle to perform your exercise.

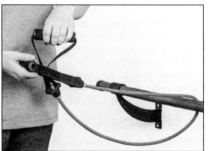

- Wrap a resistance band around a secure object such as a railing. Grasp the handles so that the band is centered around the secure object.

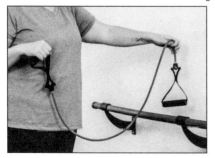

Wide-Stance Free Squat

Target: legs; hamstrings, quadriceps, glutes

1 Stand tall with a wide stance (feet more than hip-width apart) and feet slightly pointing out, arms extended down with palms in. Look straight ahead.

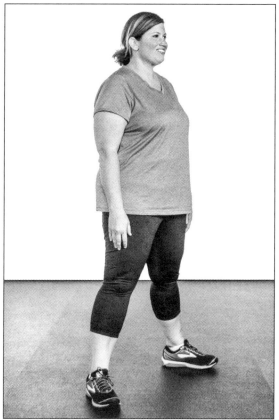

2 Inhale and slowly sit back, bending at the waist and the knees. Keep your back straight and reach the arms down toward the floor as you lower down into the squat. Be sure to sit back into the exercise and do not allow the knees to come too far over the toes (this puts strain on the knee joint rather than using your lower-body muscles).

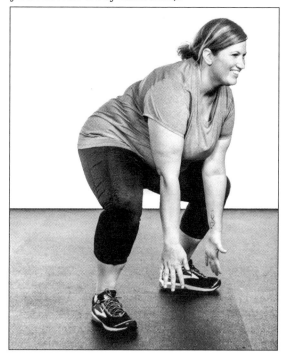

Exhale and stand back up to starting position.

Wall Push-Up

Target: chest; pectorals

1 Stand facing a wall with feet hip-width apart. Place both hands on the wall a bit wider than shoulder-width apart, with palms flat on the wall and positioned at or below the shoulders. Step back 1 to 2 feet so that you are at a bit of an incline leaning against the wall.

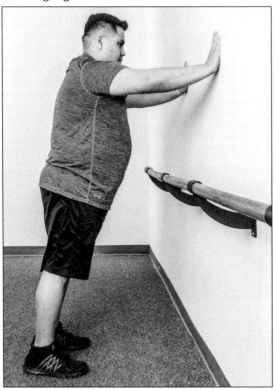

2 Inhale and bend the elbows so that you slowly lower your body towards the wall. Engage your core muscles and keep your back straight with your butt down. Stop when the elbows are at a 90-degree bend.

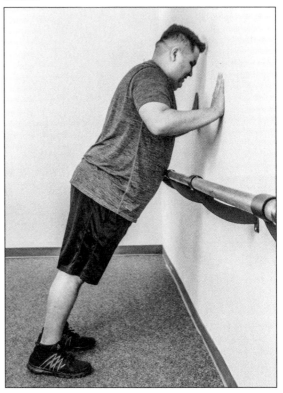

Exhale and slowly push out against the wall until arms are full extended.

NOTE: There are several progressions to this exercise. If the wall push-up is too easy, transition to an incline push-up (from a table or bed), then down to a modified push-up from your knees, and then to a full-body push-up on the floor.

Standing Row

Target: back; latissimus dorsi, trapezius, teres major and minor

1 Wrap a resistance band around a secure object. Grasp both handles of the band and step back so that you already have a good bit of resistance on the band. Stand tall with your feet hip-width apart and arms fully extended, with palms facing in while holding onto the handles. Keep the shoulders back and down. Once positioned, inhale.

2 Exhale and slowly pull the arms back, squeeze the shoulder blades and continue until the hands are positioned right below the chest. Be sure to keep your core engaged (i.e., pull the belly button in toward your spine) while performing this exercise.

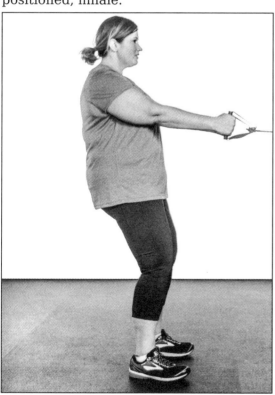

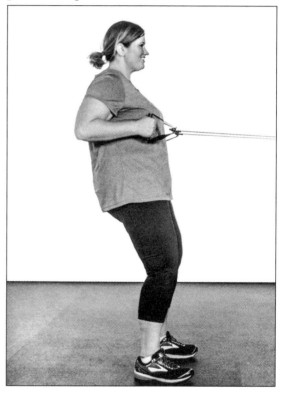

Inhale and release the arms back to their starting position.

NOTE: You can also perform this exercise from a seated position.

Plank Lift

Target: core; abdominals, obliques, low back

1 Position your hands on a mat shoulder-width apart. Be sure your elbows and hands are stacked directly underneath your shoulders. Step back so that your body is in a full plank position: up on your toes with feet flexed, back straight, slight bend in the knees, and butt down. Engage your abdominals, glutes, quadriceps, and low back muscles. Do not let your back sway. Inhale.

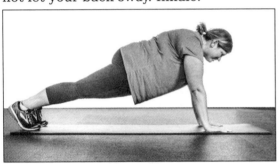

2 Exhale and slowly lower your knees down until they touch the floor.

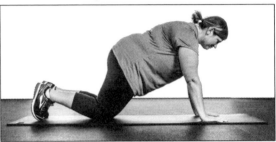

Inhale and use your core muscles to lift back up into a full plank.

Lying Hip Abduction

Target: hips; abductors

1 Lie on your left side with legs extended and stacked on top of one another. Position your left arm under your head so that you can relax your head into your hand. Inhale.

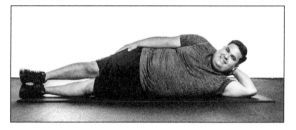

2 Exhale and slowly lift the right leg up until it is about 6 to 10 inches or 45 degrees away from the bottom leg.

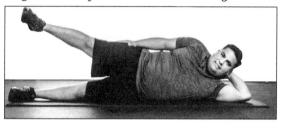

Slowly return the right leg back to starting position. Repeat for the full number of repetitions.

Turn over and repeat on the opposite side.

Lying Hip Adduction

Target: hips; adductors

1 Lie on your left side with the left leg extended. Bring the right leg over the left so that the right knee is bent and the foot is flat on the ground in front of the left leg. Position your left arm under your head so that you can relax your head into your hand. Inhale.

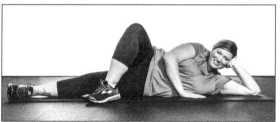

2 Exhale and slowly lift the left leg up until it's about 4 to 6 inches or 30 degrees away from the floor.

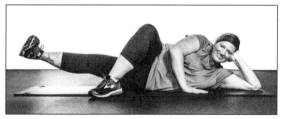

Slowly return the left leg back to starting position. Repeat for the full number of repetitions.

Turn over and repeat on the opposite side.

Single-Leg Calf Raise

Target: calves; gastrocneumius, soleus

1 Stand facing a wall or secure object. Place your hands on wall and wrap one foot around the back lower half of the opposite leg. Inhale.

2 Exhale and slowly lift up onto your toe.

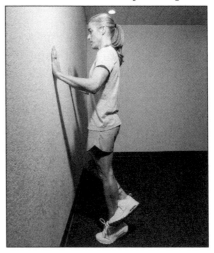

Inhale and slowly return to the starting position.

Repeat on opposite leg.

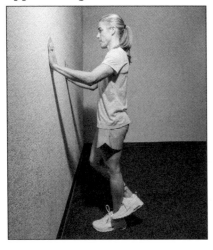

Knee Taps

Target: core; rectus abdominis

1 Lie on your back with knees bent and feet flat on the floor. Extend the arms so that your hands are palms down and in contact with your thighs. Inhale.

2 Exhale and slowly lift the upper body up, bringing your head and shoulders off the ground and moving your hands up toward the tops of your knees.

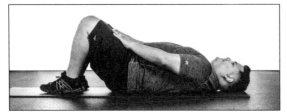

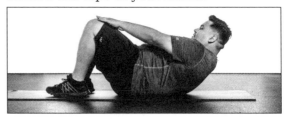

Inhale and slowly release back to the starting position.

Standing Biceps Curl

Target: arms; biceps

1 Grasp each handle of a resistance bad and stand on the band with both feet. Stand tall with your feet hip-width apart and arms fully extended, palms forward, while holding onto each handle of the band. Inhale.

2 Exhale and slowly curl your arms up toward your shoulders until they are fully flexed with knuckles up.

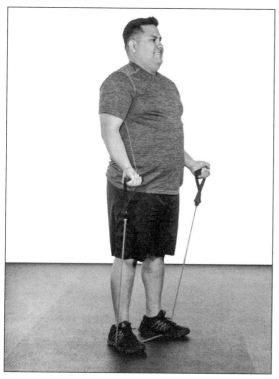

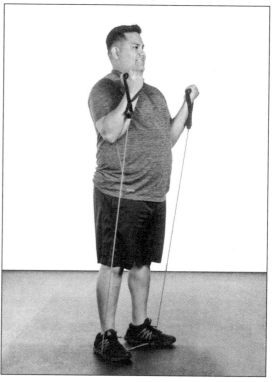

Inhale and resist the tension of the band by slowly return the arms back to starting position.

NOTE: If the resistance band has too much tension standing on it with both feet, you can drop it down to one foot to ease the resistance. If you are standing on the band with one foot, be sure to stagger your stance, with the foot that is holding the band in front of the opposite foot.

Triceps Extension

Target: arms; triceps

1 Wrap a resistance band around a secure object. Grasp the handles of the band and step back so that you already have a good bit of resistance on the band. Stand tall with your feet hip-width apart and pull the arms back so that your elbows are bent at 90 degrees and pinned at your sides with palms facing down. Inhale.

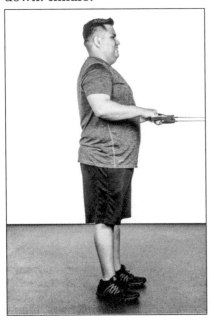

2 Exhale and slowly push the handles of the band down until the arms are near full extension. Be sure to keep the elbows pinned at your sides and do not move the shoulders during this exercise; the elbows are the only moving joint.

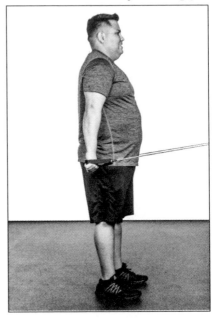

Inhale and return to starting position.

Internal Rotation

Target: shoulder, supraspinatus, infraspinatus, teres minor, subscapularis

1 Wrap a resistance band around secure object so that one end is looped around the object and the other end is free. Grasp the free handle of the band with your left hand and stand tall with feet hip-width apart facing parallel to the band with the left side of your body closest to the attachment of the band. Position yourself so that there is tension on the band and the right elbow is pinned at your side at 90 degrees, palm facing in, and forearm in contact with the body. Inhale.

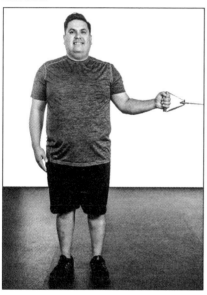

2 Exhale and slowly pull the handle in toward your waist.

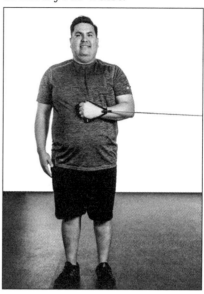

Inhale and return the arm back to starting position, maintaining a 90-degree bend throughout the range of motion. Repeat for the full number of repetitions.

Turn around, grasp handle with your right hand arm and repeat on the opposite arm.

NOTE: This exercise can also be performed with a cable machine.

External Rotation

Target: shoulder, supraspinatus, infraspinatus, teres minor, subscapularis

1 Wrap a resistance band around secure object so that one end is looped around the object and the other end is free. Grasp the free handle of the band with your right hand and stand tall with feet hip-width apart facing parallel to the band with the left side of your body closest to the attachment of the band. Position yourself so that there is tension on the band and the right elbow is pinned at your side at 90 degrees, palm facing in, and forearm in contact with the waist. Inhale.

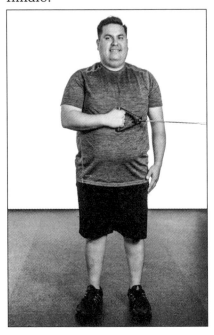

2 Exhale and slowly pull the handle out and away from the body while maintaining a 90-degree bend in the elbow.

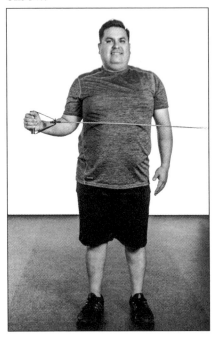

Inhale and return the arm back to starting position, maintaining a 90-degree bend in the elbow throughout the range of motion. Repeat for the full number of repetitions.

Turn around, grasp handle with right arm and repeat on the opposite arm.

NOTE: This exercise can also be performed with a cable machine.

MUSCLE SPLIT PROGRAMS

It's important not to strength train the same muscle group back to back. You need to give those muscles time to recover and rebuild; one to two days is an optimal time to allow for this muscle rebuilding and recovery to take place.

The workouts previously described here are total-body routines and thus one whole day should be left between performing these workouts (i.e., a Tuesday/Thursday or Monday/Wednesday/Friday total body workout regimen would be appropriate). If you'd rather perform muscle splits—train upper body one day and lower body another, or chest/triceps one day and back/biceps another—you can strength train on consecutive days (e.g., a Monday/Thursday upper-body and Tuesday/Friday lower-body workout regimen). Here are a few techniques to get you started with muscle split training.

Upper-body and lower-body splits. When setting up upper-body and lower-body split workouts, you'll simply train all upper body (chest, back, triceps, biceps, and shoulders) muscles on one day and then all lower body (quadriceps, hamstrings, glutes, and calves) muscles on another day. You'll generally do core (abdominal, oblique, and low back) muscles with one or both workouts. If you do core exercises for both upper and lower body workouts, be sure to leave one whole day between routines since you'll be working the core on both days. If you train the core muscles with one workout (i.e., lower body) then you can train upper body by itself the very next day.

Muscle group splits. When setting up muscle group splits, you can train each muscle group separately or couple muscle groups together. The major muscle groups include: back, biceps, chest, triceps, shoulders, legs, core. Since there are seven total major muscle groups, it is common to pair two or three muscle groups together. You can set this up to train major muscles one time or multiple times throughout the week. This all depends on how aggressive you want to be with your training and/or if you prefer to target certain muscle groups more than others (i.e., working the core muscles on multiple days). Here are some common pairing tactics to train major muscle groups:

- **Opposing muscle group splits.** This can be accomplished by pairing one muscle group with its opposing muscle group (i.e. chest and back, biceps and triceps, quadriceps and hamstrings, glutes and hip flexors, abductors and adductors, anterior and posterior deltoids, abdominals and low back). Since there several opposing muscle groups, it is common to group three different muscle groups together so that you're not strength training every day of the week.

- **Primary and assisting muscle splits.** This can be accomplished by grouping one major muscle group with its assisting muscles (i.e. chest, triceps, and shoulders).

Push and pull workouts. This can be accomplished by performing a pushing exercise (e.g., a chest press) followed by a pulling exercise (e.g., a seated row) throughout the workout; this style of training is great for an upper-body strength routine.

There are numerous ways to set up the frequency of training throughout each week. At a minimum, strength train two times per week and be sure to train each muscle group at least one time throughout the week; training each muscle group twice per week is ideal. Here are examples of how to set up the frequency of your weekly strength training:

2-Day Cycle → total body 2 x week
→ upper body 1 x week, lower body/core 1 x week
→ legs/shoulders/core 1 x week, chest/triceps/back/biceps 1 x week

3-Day Cycle → total body 3 x week
→ upper body 1 x week, core 1 x week, lower body 1 x week
→ push/pull 1 x week, core 1 x week, lower body 1 x week
→ back/biceps/core 1 x week, chest/shoulders/triceps 1 x week, legs/core 1 x week

3-day cycle rotation. This upper body/lower body strength set-up allows you to alternate weeks of more and less upper-body and strength training. Set up your workouts so that you'll do two upper-body workouts and one lower-body workout during one week and then one upper-body and two lower-body workouts the next week. Continue to alternate.

Week 1 → upper body 2 x week, lower body/core 1 x week
Week 2 → upper body 1 x week, lower body/core 2 x week

4-Day Cycle → upper body 2 x week, lower body/core 2 x week
→ chest/back 1 x week, shoulders/lower body/core 1 x week, biceps/triceps 1 x week, lower body/core 1 x week
→ push/pull 2 x week, lower body/core 2 x week
→ chest/triceps/shoulders 1 x week, back/biceps/forearms 1 x week, lower body 1 x week, core 1 x week

Mix up your strength training every four to six weeks; in other words change the format of how you're training by using some of the techniques outlined in this chapter. This will allow your body to continue to progress toward your health and fitness goals.

Chapter 6

BALANCE TRAINING

Excess weight creates both postural and biomechanical changes that directly impact physical function and ultimately balance. According to Del Porto et al. (2012), 100 percent of morbidly obese people showed abnormal postural deviations, with the most prominent changes in the spine, knees, and feet. Additionally, this excess body weight interferes with normal muscular skeletal function through physical adaptations, which leads to impaired balance, abnormal gait patterns, and increased incidence of muscle weakness—the top-three risk factors for falls.

One of the primary reasons for these physical adaptations is due to the body's shift in its center of gravity (COG) from the excess weight. This shift in COG directly affects the ability to bend, stoop, and squat, which affects balance. And when you lose weight, everything changes again, including your COG. This means that how you are used to holding your body in balance will change. Rapid weight loss, which occurs with weight-loss surgery, makes this even more challenging as it takes time for the nervous and muscular skeletal systems to catch up with bodyweight transformation. Exercise, specifically strength training combined with balance training, can speed up the process and dramatically improve your balance. There are countless ways to incorporate balance exercises into your routine. One way is to simply stand on one leg or even stagger your stance to perform an exercise. Not only will you be working the primary muscle group of the exercise, but you'll also be working the leg and ankle muscles in conjunction with the core. Another trick is to use props that create an unstable surface while performing an exercise such as a foam pad, BOSU, stability ball, aerobic step, or plyo box. Here are a few balance exercises you can try.

Single-Leg Dumbbell Biceps Curl

Target: arms; biceps and balance

1 Grasp a dumbbell in each hand and stand tall with arms extended, palms facing forward (supinated), and standing on the right leg with the left leg lifted.

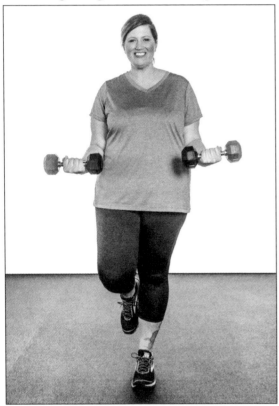

2 Slowly bring the dumbbells up until your knuckles are facing up toward the ceiling and palms are facing in toward your shoulders. Split the number of reps you're to perform with each leg (i.e., if you're going to do 12 reps, perform 6 while standing on the right leg and then 6 while standing on the left leg).

NOTE: If standing on one leg is too difficult, try staggering your stance to perform the exercise.

March in Place

Target: legs and balance

1 Stand on the foam pad with feet shoulder width apart and arms at your sides.

2 Slowly lift and bend the right knee until the right foot is lifted off the foam pad, ideally until the right thigh is parallel to the ground.

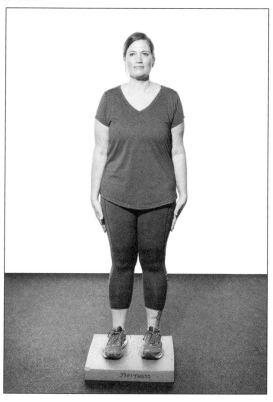

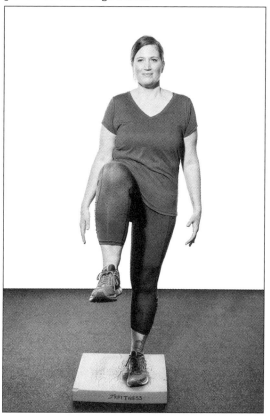

Slowly bring the right leg down to starting position and repeat with the left leg. Continue switching sides.

BOSU Dumbbell Squat

Target: legs and balance

1 Grasp a dumbbell in each hand and stand on the BOSU ball.

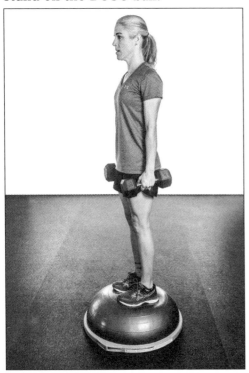

2 Inhale, engage your core, and slowly sit back into the exercise, bending at the waist and the knees. Keep your back straight and both arms positioned so that they move straight down toward your ankles.

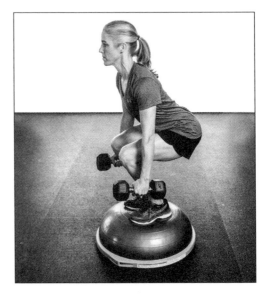

Exhale and slowly return to starting position.

NOTE: This is a challenging exercise. If you've never used the BOSU, start by positioning the BOSU next to a wall and simply try to stand on top of the BOSU (using the wall to assist in getting on as well as maintaining your balance once on the BOSU). Progress to standing on the ball without assistance from the wall, and eventually try doing different exercises, such as this one.

Stability Ball Crunch

Target: core and balance

1 Sit on top of the stability ball and then slowly walk forward so that you're positioned on the front half of the top of the ball. Place arms across your chest, round the shoulders slightly, and lean back. Keep a bend in the knees.

2 Exhale and slowly crunch forward by moving at the hips and rounding the back until your elbows come close to your thighs. Maintain a bend in the knees.

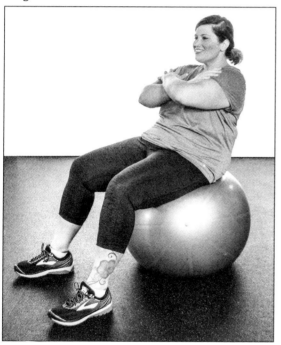

Inhale and slowly roll back into the exercise by moving at the hips and keeping the arms across your chest with shoulders rounded and chin tucked down slightly. Be careful not to arch your back and to keep a bend in the knees.

NOTE: You should feel this in your abdominal muscles and not in your low back. If you feel it in your low back, you're probably arching your back. Additionally, the ball should not be moving underneath you; keep the ball stationary throughout the movement.

Dumbbell High-Knee Step-Up

Target: legs and balance

1 Grasp a dumbbell in each hand and stand with feet shoulder-width apart in front of an aerobic step or plyo box. Inhale.

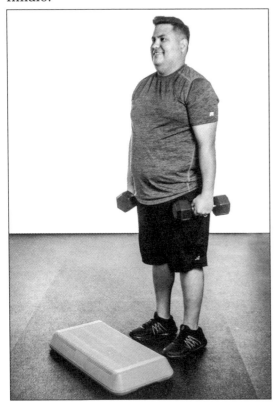

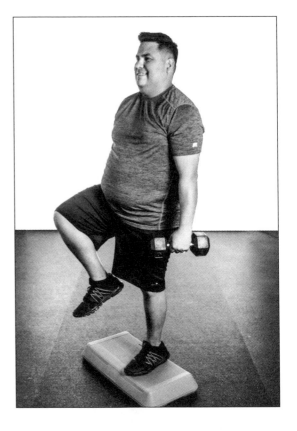

2 Exhale and step onto the box with your left foot and simultaneously bring the right knee up until the thigh is parallel to the floor. Do not let the right foot touch the box.

Slowly step back down from the box, leading with the right leg first and then the left.

Complete all repetitions and then switch sides, leading with the right leg stepping onto the step.

NOTE: Progress to a higher box or step as you become stronger and improve your balance.

Chapter 7

TESTIMONIALS

TESTIMONIAL FROM ANNIE ELMENDORF

I've struggled with my weight my entire life: gaining, losing, and gaining again—plus a little more than before—over and over again for as long as I can remember.

In the fall of 2010, I was 35 years old and weighed 275 pounds. My husband and I had a two-year-old son and planned to have another child, but I was still carrying baby weight (and then some). After considering my options, I decided to undergo gastric bypass surgery in December 2010.

My surgeon's group offered monthly support meetings for weight-loss surgery patients. At one such meeting, I met Gilbert Hernandez from JKFITNESS, who came to speak about the importance of exercise after weight-loss surgery. His message resonated with me. I decided to get more serious about fitness, and I made a standing appointment to train with Gilbert twice weekly starting a couple of months after my surgery.

The first weeks were painful, but I was committed. Before long, I was actually enjoying exercise and feeling stronger. JKFITNESS was putting together a team to train for a two-day charity bike ride. I started going on their training rides and also riding with Gilbert on the weekends.

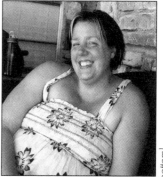

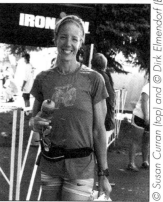

© Susan Curran (top) and © Dirk Elmendorf (bottom)

Top: Annie before. Bottom: Annie post-surgery, after finishing an Ironman race.

I'll never forget my first 20-mile training ride one hot (100° F) summer evening. We rode in the Texas Hill country just north of San Antonio. I enjoyed chatting and getting to know Julia Karlstad, the owner of JKFITNESS.

When we had our cycling team fundraiser in late summer 2011, I was just a few pounds shy of my goal weight of 160 pounds. To my surprise, Julia and Gilbert presented me with the "Rock Solid Club" award to recognize all of the hard work and positive changes that I had made in the six months I had been working with them. It was awesome!

Shortly thereafter, something funny happened. Through a lot of hard work, my body had transformed and so had my mind. I stopped thinking of myself as the fat girl and started seeing myself as the athlete I had become. On a family vacation where I didn't have access to my bike or a regular gym, I discovered that I was fit enough to run a few miles. Shockingly, I found this run to be fun.

I moved on to do a duathlon and half marathon. After the birth of my daughter in February 2013, I discovered my passion for triathlons and dabbled in several sprint- and Olympic-distance races before completing two half-Ironman-distance races in 2014. On June 28, 2015, I completed my full Ironman in Coeur D'Alene, Idaho.

At seven years post-op, I would say the surgical food "limitations" that the bariatric surgery placed on my body in order to achieve significant weight loss are minimal. In fact, as a result of my exercise, I'm able to eat extra calories and stick to a more normal diet. Today, I'm a lean, muscular, 145-pound, 42-year-old woman. I'm a wife, mother of two, competitive cyclist, and Ironman finisher. Exercising and discovering my inner athlete have been the absolute keys to my success in maintaining a healthy weight and lifestyle after weight-loss surgery.

TESTIMONIAL FROM CAROL WARYAS

In September of 2009, I walked into a gym totally convinced that it would do no good. I was a 63-year-old woman, and I had just recovered from a Roux-en-Y gastric bariatric surgery. The only reason I was there was because I had been told that unless I exercised, I would be unsuccessful at continuing to lose the weight I needed to, and more than that, keeping it off. I honestly had absolutely no hope of succeeding with exercise.

However, working with Julia Karlstad, owner and head trainer of JKFITNESS, has been the best thing I have ever done for my mind and body. She has patiently led me from dreading exercise to looking forward to it. Exercise is now the first thing that I prioritize, rather than the last thing I'd ever think about doing. Since working with Julia, I have grown in physical strength, balance, and flexibility and I have overcome numerous obstacles to my health and well-being.

I have achieved my initial goals of continuing to lose and keeping the weight off. I have progressed from "morbidly obese" when I first starting working with Julia to "obese" and now to just "overweight." Julia has helped me lose and *keep off* over 110 pounds. Now, at age 71, I'm healthier and more physically fit than I've been in years. I'm down 165 pounds from my pre-surgery weight, and I recently walked more than 25 miles over four days on a family trip.

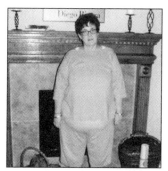

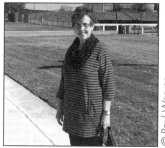

Top: Carol in 2009, just before starting with Julia. Bottom: Carol in 2017.

One of the proudest accomplishments of my life was when Julia surprised me by inducting me into her "Rock Solid Club" for my "efforts to accomplish fitness goals and improve my overall health." The reality is that I couldn't have done any of this without Julia and her belief in me, and her commitment to not let me fail. She is truly what every trainer should be but few are—a knowledgeable, trained fitness and health expert who can see beyond someone's current physical state and help them be what they should become. Her knowledge, patience, caring, guidance, and support are unsurpassed.

TESTIMONIAL FROM ELIZABETH STORIE

My weight has been up and down during my entire adult life. In fact, while in the US Army, I was unable to maintain my weight within the military standards, which ultimately forced me to leave at the age of 31 after serving eight years. I was always on a diet, but never exercised. I was a single mom, concentrating on my son's life, and gave little thought to taking care of my health and happiness. I became a nurse in 1993 and my weight spiraled out of control. In 2006 I met my husband, Ronnie, who loved me for who I was. I weighed about 180 pounds at the time, which made my BMI 35. I continued to lose and regain weight; I was 262 pounds by 2011 when my primary care doctor told me I was borderline diabetic. As a registered nurse, I cared for many patients suffering devastating effects of uncontrolled obesity, yet was in denial over the negative impact my weight was having on my own life. The news that I may become diabetic was the wake-up call I needed. It was not until 2011 that I became serious about my excess weight, and in August 2013 I had Roux-en-Y gastric bypass surgery with Dr. Pilcher in San Antonio, Texas.

I have never once regretted the decision to have surgery. I started this journey at 260 pounds, standing 61 inches (5'1")! I lost a total of 140 pounds and regained a few to reach my current set point of 135 pounds. I was a size 24-plus and am now a size 6 to 8

petite. It took me about one year to lose the weight. I had no serious medical problems post-surgery. The combination of exercise and nutrition were key to my success; but exercise was and continues to be my saving grace regarding weight loss, weight maintenance and mental stability. I want to give a big thanks to Amanda Albiar, from JKFITNESS, for physically training and motivating me to do more each week. To date, I have completed three 5Ks, a Dirty Girl 5K obstacle race, and can Zumba with the best of them—amazing for a 59-year-old with two prosthetic knees!

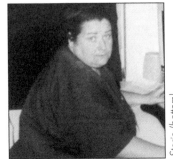

Today I am happy, healthy, and active thanks to my doctor, my dietitian, my trainer, my bariatric support group members, my husband, and myself. I love life more than ever and continue to strive to improve in all areas of life. If you are contemplating bariatric surgery or are dealing with chronic obesity, I will tell you to start slow but keep moving. If you are interested in becoming more active, make sure you are evaluated by an educated and experienced personal trainer who can adapt exercise to your fitness level and limitations.

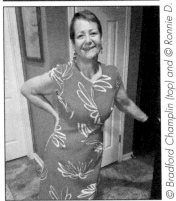

Top: Elizabeth before.
Bottom: Elizabeth post-surgery.

TESTIMONIAL FROM MARK NOBLITT

I started my journey to better health in August 2008. Tipping the scales at a whopping 500 pounds and smoking two packs of cigarettes a day, I was miserable and had been for years without even realizing it. My weight gain had happened so gradually over decades that it was out of hand before I recognized how big the problem had become. I remember even joking sarcastically about being on the "see food" diet, or about smoking, "No one likes a quitter." I lashed out at healthy eating advocates by suggesting their tips only made me want ice cream.

At age 48, I began to understand the ways in which my weight and smoking were limiting my life. Flying on airplanes was true misery (and for those poor people sitting next to me). I hated going outside nine months out of the year in South Texas because I found the heat and humidity overwhelming. Buying clothes was terrible because I was limited to the very few items in my size (60-inch waist and 5 or 6XL shirt). The time had come to find my way back to reasonably good health. After considerable research, I decided to begin my journey with gastric bypass surgery. I had tried all kinds of "diets" in the past but had just managed to yo-yo my weight. Amazingly, I've had triple-digit weight loss three times in my life!

As I've traveled my path over nearly a decade, there are some things I have learned along the way. In sharing these observations, I hope I can help others benefit from my experience.

1. Find a bariatrician in your area. They specialize in obese patients and should be able to offer a variety of surgical and nonsurgical options to get your weight loss going. Beware of docs who just advocate one procedure rather than offering you options.

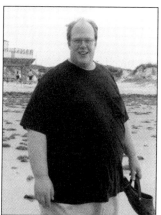

2. Set reasonable goals for yourself. Don't get overly ambitious and try to do everything all at once. For example, I was a two-pack-a-day smoker and knew I needed to knock that out before I could reasonably think about getting fit to lose weight.

3. Elicit the support of your family and friends. Tell absolutely *everyone* around you what you're doing and why. Ask them to help you in very specific ways.

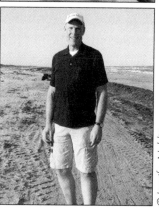

4. Plan your meals. Don't be tempted to skip meals, especially breakfast! Even if you're not a good planner, find strategies to get over this excuse for not planning your eating. Plan what you're going to eat each day and keep a food journal.

5. Get going! Do it today—not tomorrow, not on January 1, not on Monday—*today!* Don't fall into the mental trap of waiting for some milestone or until you have the perfect

Top: Mark at 500 pounds.
Bottom: Mark at 225 pounds.

plan in place. Set one goal and accomplish it while you're working out the other details. Put one foot in front of the other—get on the path and start your own journey!

TESTIMONIAL FROM NATALIE NELSON

Natalie is the cover model and fitness model throughout this book. She had the gastric sleeve procedure on August 24, 2017, and went through the largest portion of her weight loss transformation during the authorship of this book.

Natalie struggled with her weight ever since she was a child, claiming she was always chubbier than the other kids, but at 13 years old her weight really started to come on after her dad unexpectedly passed away. Natalie grew up on a farm, so activity was naturally a part of her life, but once her dad died, she stopped helping around the house or doing anything really physical. She was depressed and began to isolate herself and use food as a coping mechanism. This emotional battle over food and inactivity went on for years, and Natalie understands that bad eating habits and minimal or inconsistent exercise are what contributed to her weight gain.

Like most weight-loss surgery patients, Natalie was not new to weight-loss programs. She had tried to lose weight on several occasions, but the most she ever lost was through a medical weight loss program her mom helped enroll her in at the Mayo Clinic when she was in high school. Natalie lost forty pounds with this program, but the weight loss was temporary. She also didn't couple this program with a consistent exercise program. In fact, she never really committed to a regimented exercise plan until she started working out at JKFITNESS in 2016.

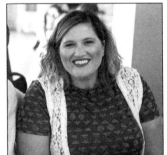

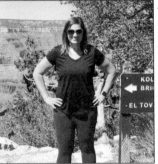

Top: Natalie before.
Bottom: Natalie after.

For years Natalie claimed she would have never considered weight-loss surgery, but In early 2017 she started to change her view. What pushed her into considering the surgery was that work was really difficult. As a registered nurse, being on her feet and shifting and moving patients all day long, she was experiencing significant pain throughout her body. "Everything hurt," as Natalie put it. She had tendonitis in her hips, plantar fasciitis in her feet, and pinched nerves in her spine that were causing severe havoc on her back. At 302 pounds, her physical health was really affecting her emotional health. Another thing that really hurt, but at the same time drove her to get serious about weight loss, was when she was home playing with her five-year-old nephew and he said, "Natalie, your fat." She wanted to be a positive role model for him. It was time to change.

After Natalie had the gastric sleeve weight-loss surgery, there were emotional highs and lows. It wasn't until she was three months post-op that she was completely confident she had made the right decision; at this point she could finally start to feel the physical and emotional benefits of the surgery. When she started her journey, she didn't believe she could lose all of the weight, but as of June 11, 2018, she's down 124 pounds, just 13 pounds shy of her goal weight. Now she feels empowered to not only achieve her goal weight, but sustain it long-term.

Natalie was inspired to make exercise a part of her weight loss journey because she wanted to be overall healthier and set an example to her friends, family, patients and coworkers. Today, Natalie literally has a new lease on life! She has fully embraced the lifestyle change that comes along with having the weight-loss surgery. Natalie enjoys sharing her story and tells everyone that this is the best thing she ever could have done for herself and her health.

TESTIMONIAL FROM TERRY DOWD

This testament was taken from an interview the author did with Terry Dowd on November 18, 2017. Terry has been a client of the author off and on over the past 10-plus years.

Terry was in the Army, a physically active profession, for several years. When he left the military in his mid-20s, he began working in sedentary jobs. Due to this reduced activity, Terry started to notice his clothes fitting tighter and having to buy larger sizes to accommodate his expanding waist line.

At his heaviest, Terry topped the scales at 413 pounds. After eight long years of trying to lose weight non-surgically, he was only able to lose about 80 pounds, despite help of a medical weight-loss professional, dieticians, and personal trainers. He tried to lose more but could never get past the 330-pound mark. Approaching 40 years of age, Terry realized his excess weight put him at a very high risk of suffering a heart attack or stroke, or as he says, "I was going to kill myself." He then made the decision to have weight-loss surgery. On December 12, 2013, the day before his 40th birthday, Terry underwent the gastric bypass weight-loss surgery procedure to improve his heart health.

The surgery was the ticket Terry needed to move past that 330-pound set point he struggled with. After the surgery, he got down to 234 pounds, losing a total of 179 pounds. While he lost a lot of weight with the surgery, exercise was paramount to Terry's success. As he says:

> "*The weight loss allowed me to be able to run again. I had not run since 1996 ... when I was in the army. I really enjoy running because it clears my mind ... it sets me free. Being able to run and do full sit-ups again gave me a sense of accomplishment that continues to motivate me. I'm also doing strength-training boot camps with Kimberly Black at JKFITNESS. She's improved my strength and muscle tone, and has dramatically improved my flexibility.*"

Terry is a designer—a very sedentary job where he sometimes sits for 10 to 14 hours at a time. This is the primary reason why he makes exercise a priority. To keep the weight off, he continues to be diligently focused on nutrition, which is also a huge component of his success. To this day, Terry has built an accountability system with fitness professionals and dieticians to ensure his health, fitness, and weight-loss goals are achieved.

RESOURCES

BIBLIOGRAPHY

Davis, Bruce. "There Are 50,000 Thoughts Standing Between You and Your Partner Every Day!" *The Huffington Post*. July 23, 2013. Accessed June 19, 2018. https://www.huffingtonpost.com/bruce-davis-phd/healthy-relationships_b_3307916.html.

Del Porto, Hannah, Celia Pechak, Darla Smith, and Rebecca Reed-Jones. "Biomechanical Effects of Obesity on Balance." *International Journal of Exercise Science* 5, no. 4 (2012): 301–20.

Horowitz, Sala. "Health Benefits of Meditation: What the Newest Research Shows." *Alternative and Complementary Therapies* 16, no. 4 (August 3, 2010): 223–28, accessed July 14, 2017, doi: 10.1089/act.2010.16402.

Rama, Swami. "The Real Meaning of Meditation." *Yoga International*, June 3, 2013, accessed July 16, 2017. https://yogainternational.com/article/view/the-real-meaning-of-meditation.

Segal, Zindel V., J. Mark G. Williams, and John D. Teasdale. *Mindfulness-Based Cognitive Therapy for Depression: A New Approach to Preventing Relapse*. New York: Guilford Press, 2002.

Tigunait, Pandit Rajmani. "What Is Meditation?" *Yoga International*, October 17, 2014, accessed September 4, 2017. https://yogainternational.com/article/view/what-is-meditation.

Tolle, Eckhart. *The Power of Now: A Guide to Spiritual Enlightenment*. Novato, CA: New World Library, 1999.

ADDITIONAL RESOURCES

Yoga:

www.bodypositiveyoga.com

www.yogajournal.com

Myofascial release:

www.tptherapy.com

The Mindful Diet: How to Transform Your Relationship with Food for Lasting Weight Loss and Vibrant Health by Ruth Wolever, Ruth, Beth Reardon, and Tania Hannan (New York: Scribner, 2015).

Mindful Eating: A Guide to Rediscovering a Healthy and Joyful Relationship with Food by Jan Chozen Bays (Boulder, CO: Shambhala Publications, Inc., 2017).

The Roll Model: A Step-by Step Guide to Erase Pain, Improve Mobility, and Live Better in Your Body by Jill Miller (Las Vegas, NV: Victory Belt Publishing, 2014).

INDEX

ACKNOWLEDGMENTS

I have a tendency to get involved in many undertakings at one time, and this book was no exception. But being busy is what drives me—I love feeling accomplished! As I wrote this book, I continued to own and operate my business, personally train and motivate clients, mentor and manage my staff, be a friend, be involved in the community, be a spouse, and be a mom. With a short timeline to produce the manuscript of this book, I can say without question that it wouldn't have been possible without the help of many. And for many I am thankful!

First and foremost, I thank God for giving me the drive and motivation to write another book. I thank my family, especially my wife, Audrey, for her love and support and for sacrificing quality time together while I wrote this book. My young son, Jackson, and baby daughter, Madison, both gave me strength and courage to keep pushing through to finish this book.

To my parents, Dennis and Carolyn Karlstad, thank you for your unwavering love and encouragement and for building the foundation of my work ethic. To my sister, Heather Anderson, and her family, Joe Anderson, Cheyanne Luther, and Dakota Luther for the positive encouragement.

A tribute to Bryan Nguyen, my photographer, for going the extra mile and working countless hours to create the best pictures for my book. And a special thanks to the models in my book: Natalie Nelson, Matthew Martinez, and Tumay Nguyen.

To Carol Waryas, Annie Elmendorf, Elizabeth Storie, Mark Noblitt, Natalie Nelson, and Terry Dowd—thank you for sharing your personal stories as testaments to the importance of exercise in the surgical weight-loss journey.

I am honored to have had the opportunity work with many health professionals over the years. The collaboration helped me expand my knowledge of the bariatric patient. Special thanks to Laurel Dierking, who contributed to Chapter 1 of this book.

Thank you Kathy O'Brien and Carol Waryas for giving me insight into the process of working with a publisher. To the publishing professionals at Ulysses Press for their dedication in working with me to edit and publish this book—thank you! A salute to Leslie Luttrell for giving me legal guidance in this project.

I'm forever grateful for my JKFITNESS team! I am also indebted to all of my clients, who not only gave me experience in the field over the years but also helped keep me accountable throughout this project. I have witnessed numerous individuals make the change of the lifetime and I hope this book inspires many more to do the same! You are the reason I continue to do what I do.

ABOUT THE AUTHOR AND CONTRIBUTOR

Julia Karlstad, M.Ed., CSCS, SFN-ISSA, has more than 13 years of experience developing, implementing, and directing exercise, education, and training programs within medically-based programs and facilities. In 2008, she founded JKFITNESS, a personal training and wellness studio that specializes in weight-loss programs. Combined, JKFITNESS completes 600-plus hours of personal training each month. Julia has personally worked with thousands of clients, many of whom were weight-loss surgery patients.

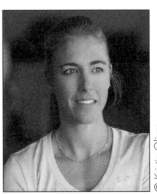
© Kristin Oliver

Julia has a master's of education in exercise science from Auburn University of Montgomery as well as a bachelor's of science in basic sciences from the United States Air Force Academy. She is the author of *Rx Fitness for Weight Loss: The Medically Sound Solution to Get Fit and Save Your Life,* a book that is specifically about exercise as it relates to weight loss. She has also been published in numerous periodicals, a motivational speaker for countless organizations, and was featured with one of her clients on TLC's *My 600 Pound Life* reality show.

Laurel Dierking, M.Ed., NFPT, 500YTT, who contributed to the mindfulness and meditative practice sections in Chapter 1, is a health and fitness professional with extensive hands-on experience in yoga and individualized wellness training. She focuses on improving the connection to the self through mindful movement, body awareness, gratitude, and compassion.